LEUCODERMA

Diseases of White Patches

(Second Edition)

By the Same Author:

- **Textbook of Dermatology**
- **Comprehensive Dermatology and Sexually Transmitted Diseases**
- **Textbook of Dermatology for Homeopaths (English and Spanish Edition)**
- **Illustrated Textbook of Dermatology**
- **Skin and Hair in Health and Disease (English and Hindi Edition)**
- **MCQ in Dermatology and Venereology**
- **Can We Cure Psoriasis?**

LEUCODERMA

Diseases of White Patches

(Second Edition)

Dr Ramji Gupta
MD (AIIMS)
Senior Consultant and Professor of Dermatology
Indraprastha Apollo Hospital
New Delhi

Formerly at
Department of Dermatology
All India Institute of Medical Sciences
New Delhi

PEEPEE
PUBLISHERS AND DISTRIBUTORS (P) LTD.

LEUCODERMA
Diseases of White Patches

Published by
Pawaninder P. Vij and Anupam Vij
Peepee Publishers and Distributors (P) Ltd.
Head Office: 160, Shakti Vihar, Pitam Pura
Delhi-110034 (India)

Correspondence Address:
7/31, First Floor, Ansari Road
Daryaganj, New Delhi-110002 (India)
Ph: 65195868, 23246245, 9811156083
e-mail: peepee160@yahoo.co.in, peepee160@rediffmail.com
peepee160@gmail.com
Website: www.peepeepub.com

First Edition : 2012
Second Edition : 2016

ISBN: 978-81-8445-186-3

This book is dedicated to
my parents,
wife
and children

PREFACE TO THE SECOND EDITION

In this new and revised edition, the text has been revised and updated. Many color photographs have also been added. Few color photographs which were not up-to-date were replaced.

Comments and criticisms are always welcome to improve the book.

Ramji Gupta

PREFACE TO THE FIRST EDITION

In spite of tremendous amount of research in the field of leucoderma (vitiligo) during the last few decades, most patients and general public still consider that leucoderma is an incurable disease. This is probably due to the lack of knowledge and paucity of literature available to general public, especially patients. The development of pigmentation or improvement in leucoderma patches depends upon the selection of proper treatment regimen and the presence of reasonable number of viable melanocytes (the cells which produce pigment) in the leucoderma patch. Every patient should know that leucoderma is basically a harmless disease. The patients having leucoderma are as efficient in physical, intellectual and sexual terms as any other normal person.

This book aims to present various kinds of clinical presentation and modalities of treatment for the knowledge of patients and general public. It is also useful to general physicians, postgraduate (medical) students and knowledge-hungry dermatologists.

Comments and criticism are welcome for improving the contents of this book.

Ramji Gupta

ACKNOWLEDGEMENTS

I thank Dr (Mrs) Sachi Gupta for going through the manuscript critically and correcting it by page to page. Thanks are due to Dr Sameer Gupta and Dr Charu Gupta of Philadelphia, USA, Dr Sarthak Gupta and Dr Saima of Meryland, USA, for their healthy criticism and suggestions.

A special thanks to Mr Pawaninder P Vij, Director, Peepee Publishers and Distributors (P) Ltd., and his team specially Mr Pawan Sharma for his all-round support.

This book would have not completed without the moral support of my wife, Mrs Saroj Gupta.

Ramji Gupta

CONTENTS

CHAPTER

1 Leucoderma: An Introduction

Leucoderma is a term generally used for white patches present on the skin and mucous membranes (lips and genitals). This disease has afflicted the mankind since time immemorial and general population often confuse it with leprosy. This is perhaps the reason why patients having leucoderma have to suffer the humiliation of this stigma. Leucoderma manifests with white patches on the skin. However, all white patches on the skin are not leucoderma. It is generally considered to be incurable. With the tremendous progress during the last few years, leucoderma can now be considered to be a completely curable disease.

Leucoderma (vitiligo) is basically a harmless disease except for its cosmetic implication. Each and every patient must be made aware of this fact. There are no risks from leucoderma to any of the internal organs as compared to diabetes mellitus, hypertension etc. There is no need for any inhibitions and prohibitions. A patient of leucoderma can be as efficient physically, intellectually and sexually as any other individual. In fact there is no justification for even treating this disease if the patient and the society are ready to accept this change in the skin, as we do not discriminate animals when they have white spots/patterns of different colors/shades on their skin (Fig.1.1).

The main approach for the treatment of this disease has been directed towards inducing repigmentation in the white areas, while almost no effort has been made to control the disease process. The latter should be the first priority because if this is not done, the

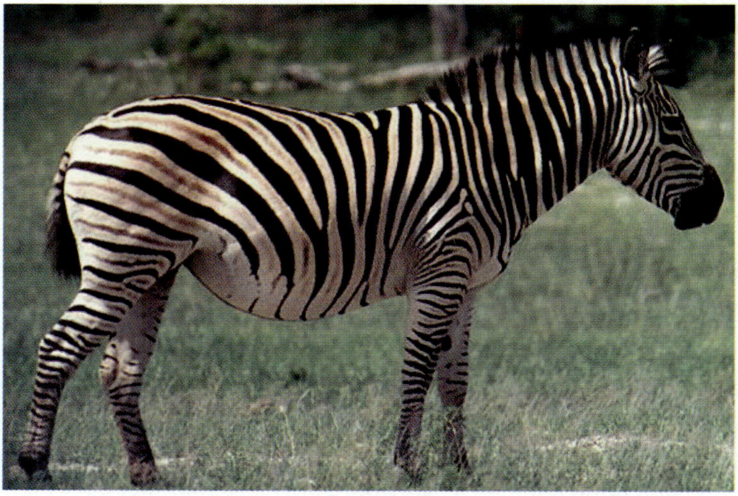

Fig. 1.1

patient will continue to develop new lesions even while the old lesions are getting repigmented. This is commonly the major cause of frustration in the patients as well as in the doctors.

Once the activity of the disease is controlled adequately many patients start showing spontaneous repigmentation of the existing lesions even without any additional treatment. In case, if the rate of repigmentation is slow or if some of the lesions do not repigment at all or if it is desired to have a quicker recovery, the patient should be given additional treatment for inducing the repigmentation at a faster rate. This can be continued till either all the areas have become repigmented or there is no further improvement for a period of at least 4-6 months. Such residual white spots can either be left alone or subjected to surgical treatment depending upon the requirement of the patients.

In this way almost every patient having leucoderma can be treated completely as per his or her requirement.

CHAPTER 2

Normal Color of the Skin and its Formation

The color of the normal human skin is decided by the melanin and the carotenoids present in the epidermis (outer layer of the skin) and oxidized and reduced hemoglobin in the dermis (inner layer of the skin). Among these pigments, melanin is the main pigment that determines the skin color of an individual. In human, there are two types of melanin pigment. The first one which decides the skin color, is genetically determined and is responsible for the amount of melanin pigment in the individual, while the second one consists of the pigmentation due to exposure to sunlight or to other substances. Melanin is synthesize in special structure called melanocyte. These specialize cells are present in basal (inner most) layer of the epidermis. Melanocytes constitute about 10 percent of the cells in the basal layer.

After melanin is synthesized in the melanocytes it is transferred to the keratinocytes (another layer of cells above the basal layer) and finally thrown out with the loss of the stratum corneum (outermost layer of the skin).

CHAPTER

3 Causes of Leucoderma

The cause of leucoderma varies in different patients. In a group of patients in whom leucoderma spreads very fast, the areas tend to become generalize and are usually distributed equally on both sides of the body (bilaterally symmetrical). Such cases are believed to be caused by auto-immune mechanism, where the immunity of one's own body progressively destroys the melanocytes, leading to depigmentation. This is presently the most commonly accepted cause of leucoderma. It has been possible to demonstrate the presence of specific circulating auto-antibodies to melanocyte cell surface antigen and its level to the extent of depigmentation along with demonstration of lymphocytic infiltration in the dermis and epidermis of leucoderma. In addition, a proportion of the leucoderma patients show the presence of non-specific auto-antibodies, such as anti-nuclear antibodies, anti-thyroid antibodies, anti-parietal cell antibodies, anti-microsomal antibodies and less commonly, other types of auto-antibodies suggesting that leucoderma is an auto-immune disease.

In some patients the lesions are localised to an area corresponding to a nerve segment and are strictly limited to one side of the body (unilateral). These cases are called 'segmental leucoderma' and are presumed to be due to neurogenic factors released from the nerve endings which are toxic to melanocytes.

In another group of patients, melanocytes are suppose to be destroyed due to a defect in self-protective mechanism that removes toxic substances. Such group of patient includes patients with halo

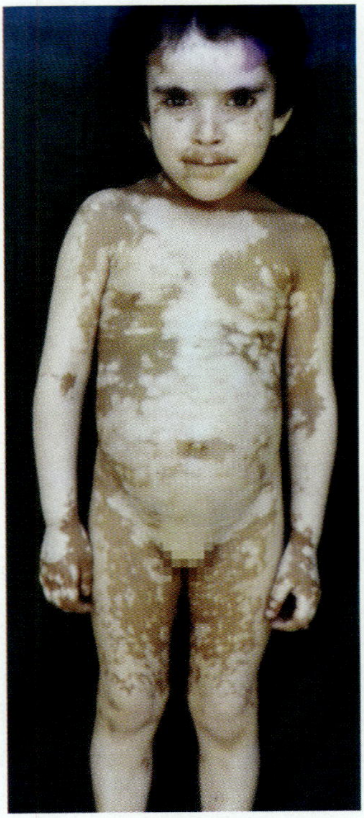

Fig. 3.1: Generalized Leucoderma–child

naevus which consists of a zone of de-pigmented skin (halo) around a pigmented mole, indicating that the body is trying to destroy the pigmented mole. The pigmented mole in such patients tends to become progressively smaller till it disappears completely. During this period the patient may develop leucoderma lesions elsewhere on the body as well.

However, after the pigmented mole has been completely destroyed, the leucoderma lesions also tend to disappear or reduce substantially. Patients having malignant melanoma (a type of cancer) have been seen to develop extensive de-pigmentation of the skin, which is based on the same phenomenon that destroys the melanocytes extensively.

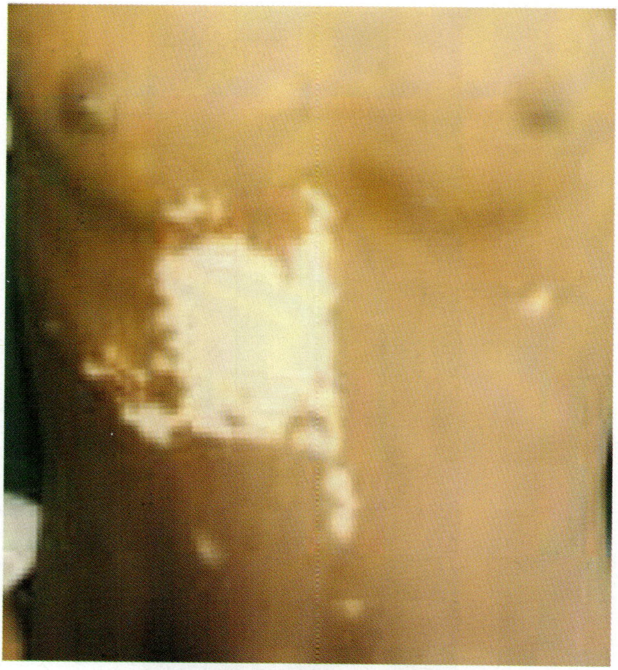

Fig. 3.2: Segmental Leucoderma

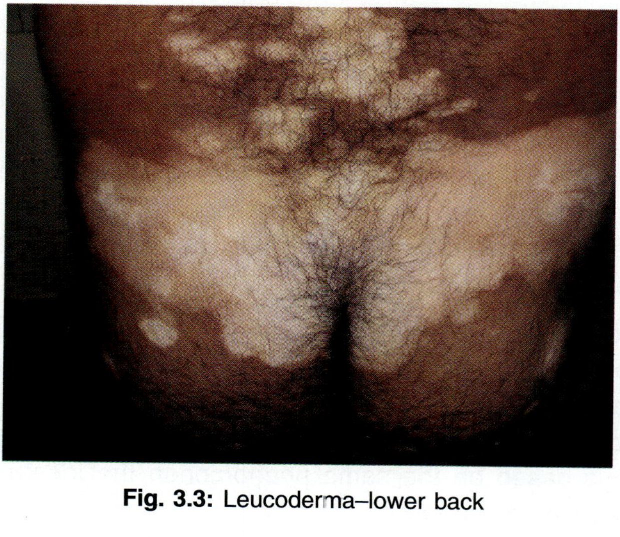

Fig. 3.3: Leucoderma–lower back

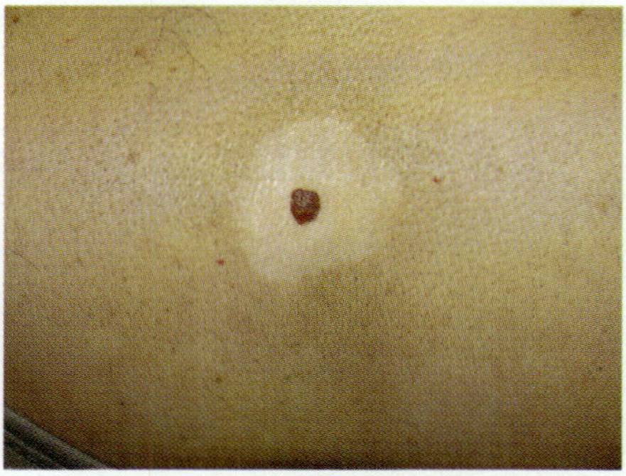

Fig. 3.4: Halo nevus

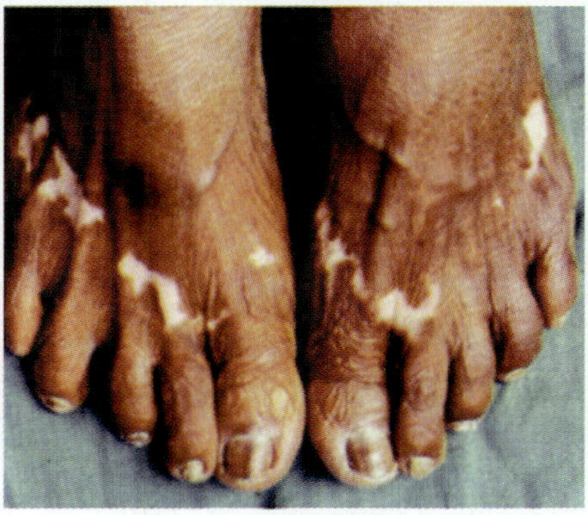

Fig. 3.5: Leucoderma due to chappal

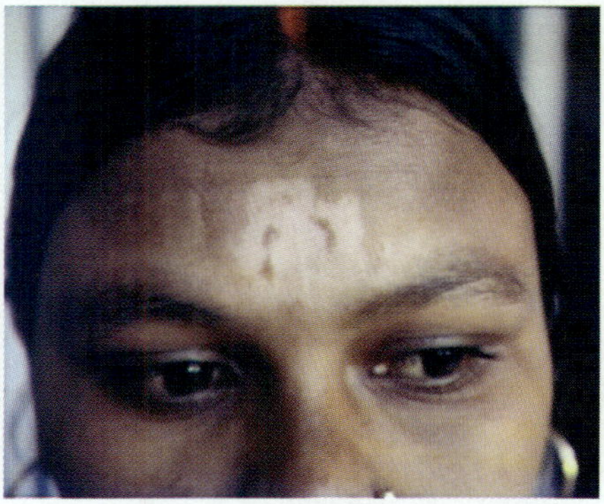

Fig. 3.6: Leucoderma due to bindi

In some cases, leucoderma develops in the skin areas which come in contact with plastic or rubber articles.

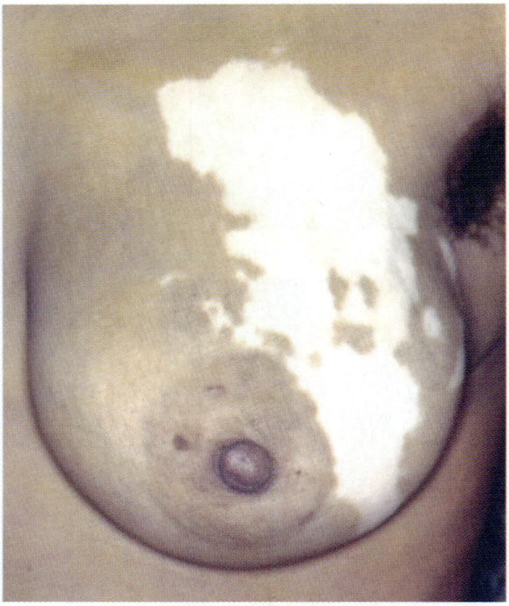

Fig. 3.7: Leucoderma on the breast due to a purse

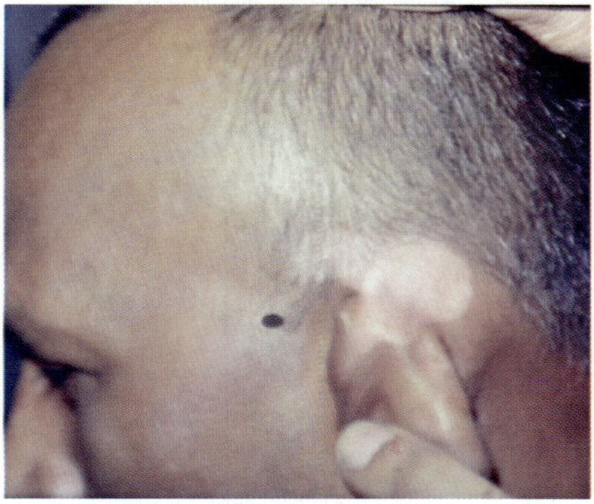

Fig. 3.8: Leucoderma–post auricular area due to spectacle frame

Slippers can cause leucoderma on the feet; gloves on the hands; plastic bindis on the central part of the forehead; purse kept under the brassieres can produce leucoderma on the upper part of the breast and so on. Such lesions are due to the action of certain phenolic compounds, such as monobenzyl ether of hydroquinone or paratertiary butyl phenol, which are used as accelerators and anti-oxidants in the manufacturing of plastics and rubber. Such chemicals, if present in the finished product, can cause leucoderma if they penetrate the skin and destroy the pigment producing cells i.e. melanocytes. In some cases, leucoderma remains limited to the areas coming in contact with the rubber or the plastic article(s), but in other cases, leucoderma lesions can appear in other areas as well. Some of the workers employed in plastic or rubber industries have been seen to develop leucoderma locally and sometimes even generalized leucoderma. Stoppage of further exposure to plastic and rubber articles usually stop the progression of the disease and may lead to repigmentation of the skin in some cases, even without any treatment. Continued exposure, however, is expected to worsen the disease.

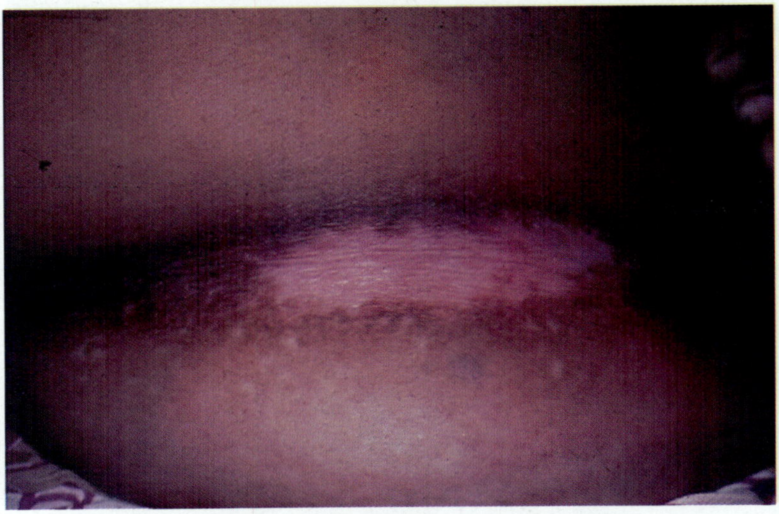

Fig. 3.9: Leucoderma waist due to pressure of petticoat string

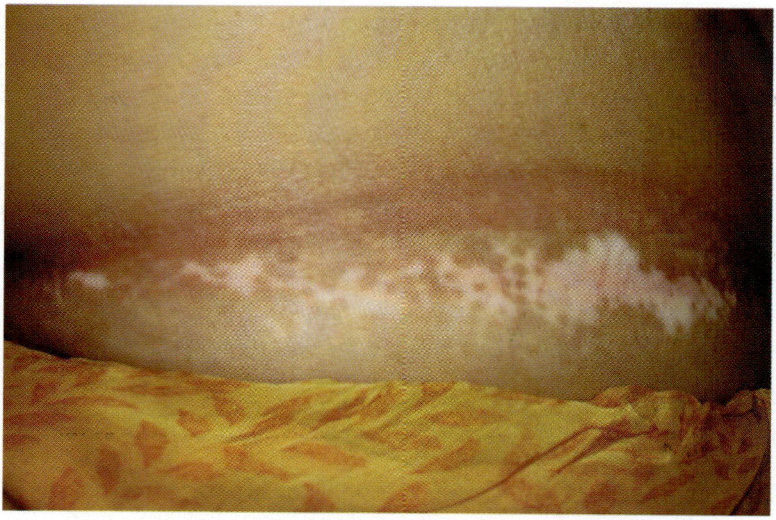

Fig. 3.10: Leucoderma waist on treatment–appearance of pigmentation

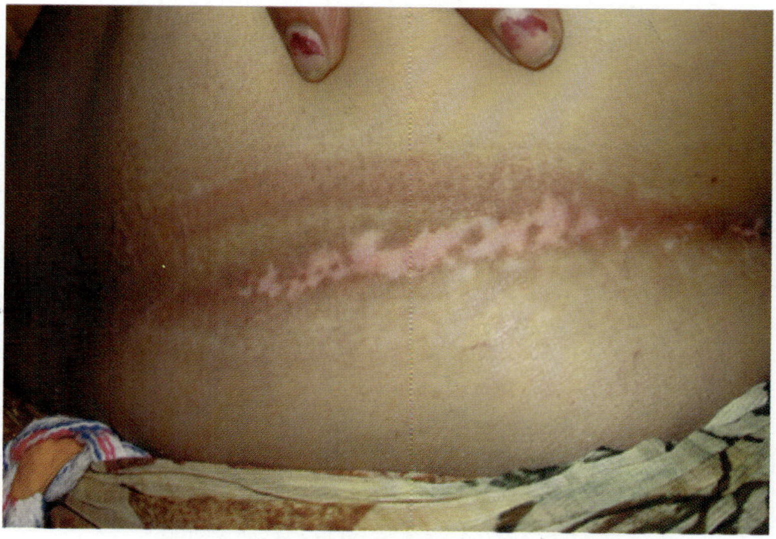

Fig. 3.11: Leucoderma waist–on treatment

Leucoderma has been seen on the flanks of some women who tie their petticoat or salwar very tightly. This is probably due to prolong pressure of the string, which interferes with the formation of pigment by the melanocytes. Similar pressure from elastic bands in socks, brassieres, etc. can also lead to leucoderma in respective areas. If further pressure is avoided by putting a very thick layer of cloth between the string and the skin, the leucoderma lesions in some of the cases may be avoided.

Some individuals have the tendency to develop leucoderma in response to minor trauma. In such patients leucoderma is seen on the knees, elbows, ankles, knuckles and other areas that are prone to repeated trauma. Some of these patients may have linear lesions of leucoderma corresponding to the line of scratches. Similarly, sports

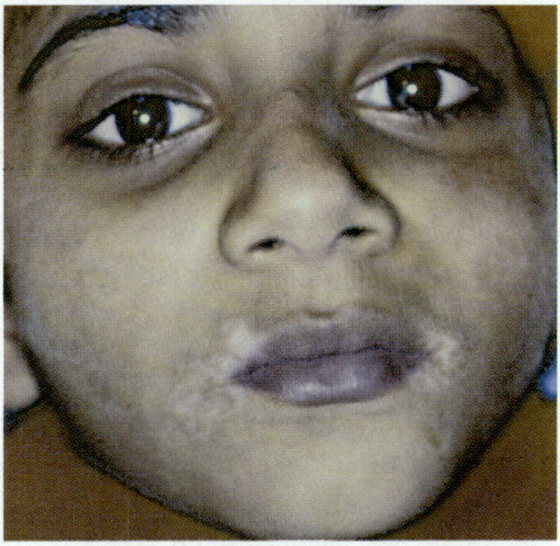

Fig. 3.12: Leucoderma–after herpes simplex

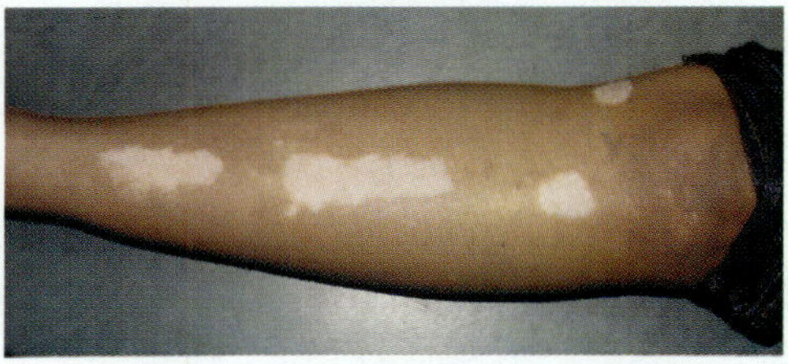

Fig. 3.13: Leucoderma–on scratch marks (Koebner's phenomenon)

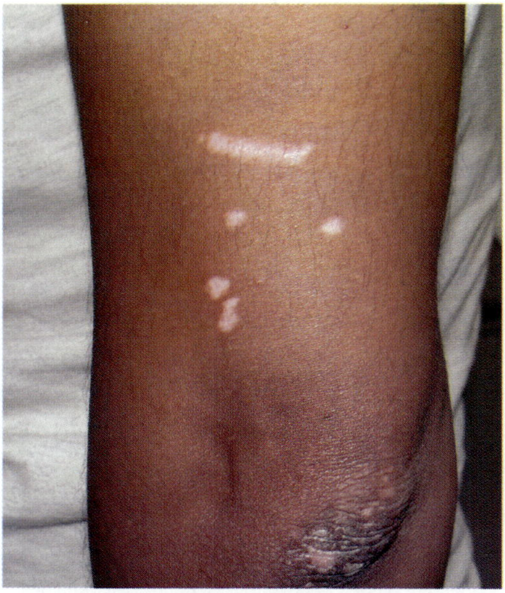

Fig. 3.14: Leucoderma on scratch marks-arm

persons may develop leucoderma on the front of their legs and other trauma-prone sites. Mosquito bites or other types of skin lesions can also leave behind depigmented spots.

In many cases, however, the cause of leucoderma is still not known. Even when the leucoderma are located at specific sites, the areas of lesions often develop at other sites, suggesting that leucoderma may be caused by a variety of agents, some of which are known, while others are still not known. However, leucoderma is a single disease entity caused by multiple factors. All factors, however, do not operate in all the cases.

FAMILIAL TENDENCY

Occurrence of leucoderma in more than one member in some families suggests that there is a genetic predisposition for the development of leucoderma.

However, a positive family history is only found in about 10-30% of the cases. Since leucoderma is more often present in the distant relatives, the frequency with which a positive family history is elicited depends on how well informed the patient is about his relatives and how carefully the doctor has taken the history.

SOCIAL STIGMA

Social stigma has always been attached to leucoderma in all classes of society in all ages. School children are often teased by their friends and may be discriminated against even by ill-informed teachers. Patients sometimes may be stared at by strangers and are often offered unsolicited advice and different ways to cure the disease. The greatest social difficulty posed by leucoderma is marriage. It is rare to find a family that will accept a person having leucoderma. The individual may have to compromise on educational abilities and social standing of the partner in order to find a willing mate. Siblings, children and even other relatives of leucoderma patients may have difficulty in getting married and this places a burden of guilt on the patient. When leucoderma develops after marriage, the reactions are usually not as intense especially if there are children and the marriage has lasted for a significant period.

During matrimonial alliances, if some relative is found to have leucoderma, a question is often raised whether the matrimonial candidate is likely to develop leucoderma in later life or whether there would be an increase tendency in their children to develop leucoderma. Since direct transmission of leucoderma is extremely rare, the risk involved in such instances seems to be very insignificant.

CHAPTER

4 Clinical Presentation

Leucoderma presents as asymptomatic areas that are mostly depigmented (white) but may be hypopigmented (less white). There is no other change like scaling, atrophy, loss of hair, loss of sweating or loss of sensation in the area. The disease can start at any age between childhood to old age, and occasionally it may even be seen in newborn babies. Leucoderma involves both the sexes equally. There is no known racial variation in the prevalence of leucoderma.

The disease occurs all over the world and affects almost every community and nationality irrespective of the color or type of skin. It is estimated that approximately 0.5-1 percent of the world population suffers from leucoderma, though certain communities are known to have a higher incidence of this disease. Assuming a population of 1200 million in India, about 6-12 million people in our country are probably affected by the disease.

The onset of leucoderma, at times, may not be noticed initially because the lesions are asymptomatic and may be located on inconspicuous areas of the body. In a large majority of patients, leucoderma starts as a single lesion. Further course of the disease varies in different patients.

Some patients may develop just few more lesions over the next several months or years and there may be only a mild increase in the size of the initial lesions. In a small proportion of these patients, a few episodes of relatively faster activity occur. In another small group, after the initial slow progression, the disease may become static or there may even be a spontaneous repigmentation of the lesions. In another group of patients, the disease may progress at a much faster rate from the very onset or after an initial slow progression. Such patients usually develop several new lesions and extensive disease within a period of few months. Such progression, however, is only seen rarely. The slowly progressive leucoderma leading to extensive involvement, however, is not uncommon. The degree of loss of pigmentation varies in different lesions.

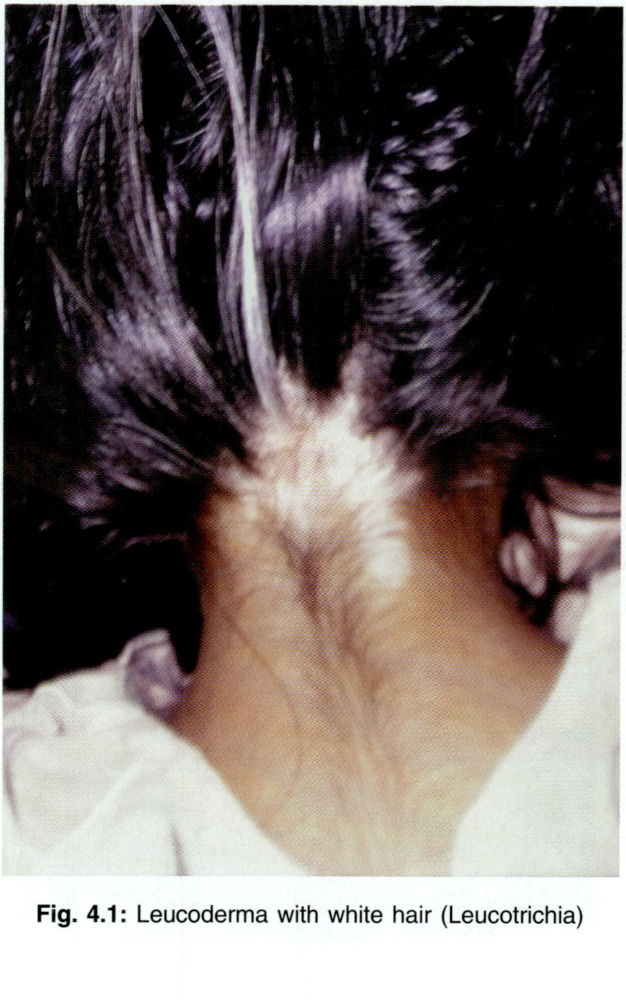

Fig. 4.1: Leucoderma with white hair (Leucotrichia)

There may be a faint hypopigmentation or complete depigmentation or varying shades between the two poles.

The hypopigmentation usually becomes more pronounced gradually till the lesion becomes completely depigmented, but sometimes in the same patch there may be areas of different degree of hypopigmentation. Such lesions are called trichrome leucoderma. Some of the lesions may have islands of normal color skin and occasionally it may become difficult to ascertain whether this is the uninvolved area or it is the repigmented skin following therapy.

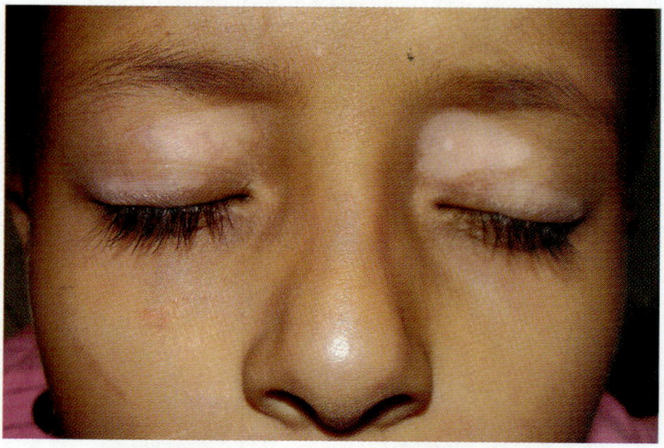

Fig. 4.2: Leucoderma–upper eyelid

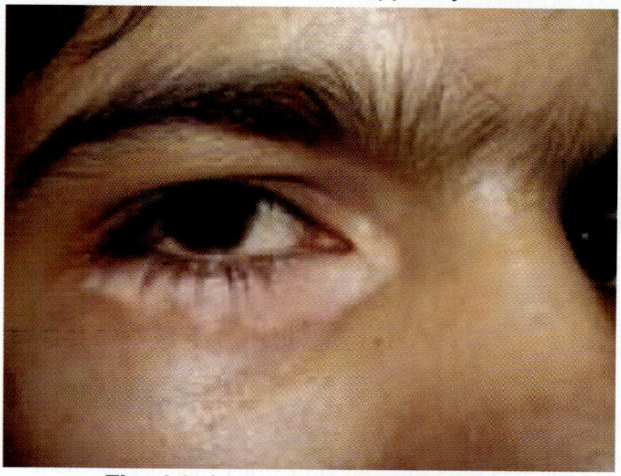

Fig. 4.3: Leucoderma–lower eyelid

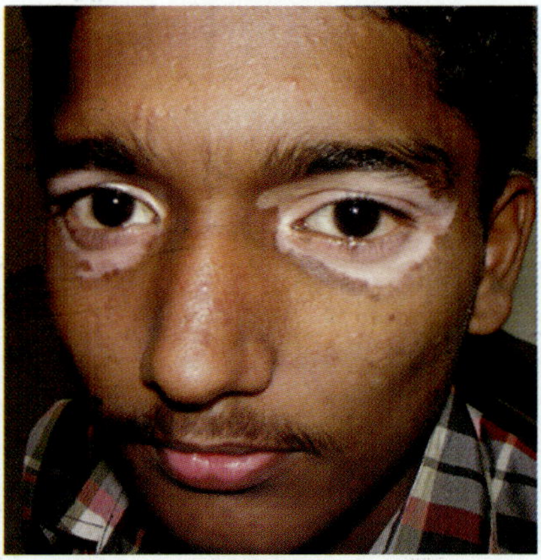

Fig. 4.4: Leucoderma–around eye

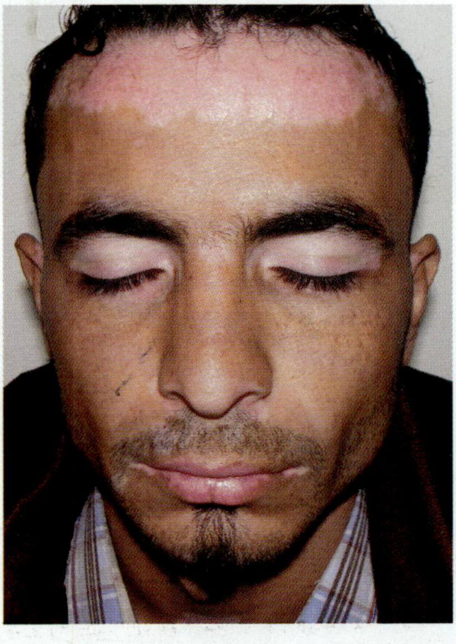

Fig. 4.5: Leucoderma–forehead, upper eyelid and lips

Presence of a slightly hyperpigmented area suggests that the area is a repigmented skin.

In case the area is located on a hairy region, the hair may also lose their pigment and become white. This is called *leucotrichia*. There is however, no relationship between the greying of hair due to old age or premature grey hair (canities) and leucoderma. The size of leucoderma lesions varies from 1-2 mm to very large areas covering

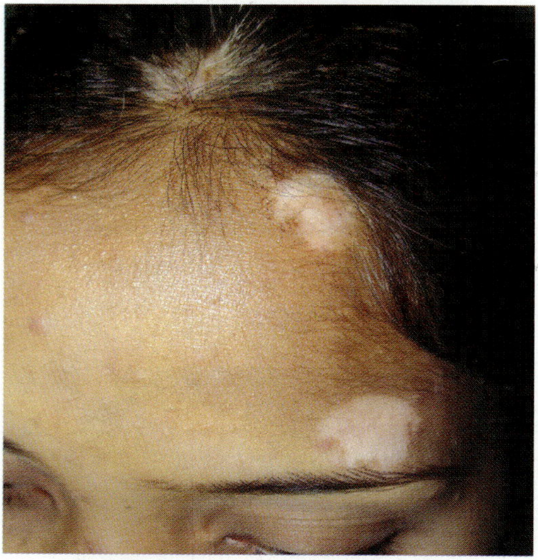

Fig. 4.6: Leucoderma–forehead

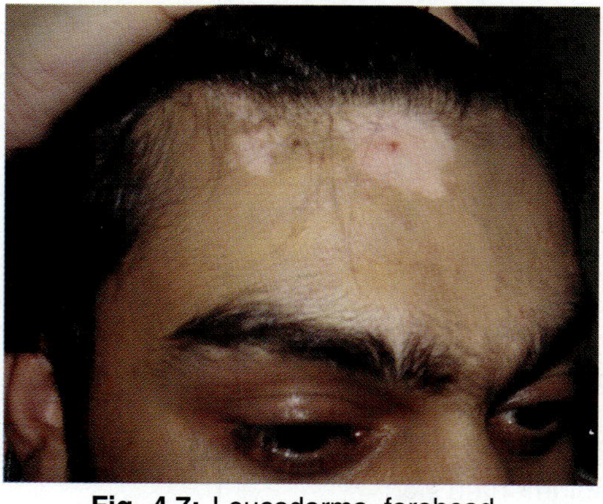

Fig. 4.7: Leucoderma–forehead

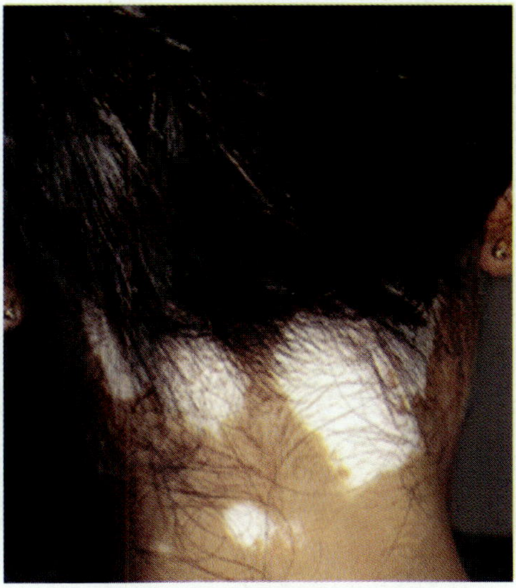

Fig. 4.8: Leucoderma–neck

almost the whole limb, trunk or even the entire body. The number of the lesions can vary from a single lesion to multiple lesions. The shapes of the lesions are variable; they may be round, oval or irregular. The location of the lesions also varies in different patients. Almost any site may be involved but generally, the face, the extremities

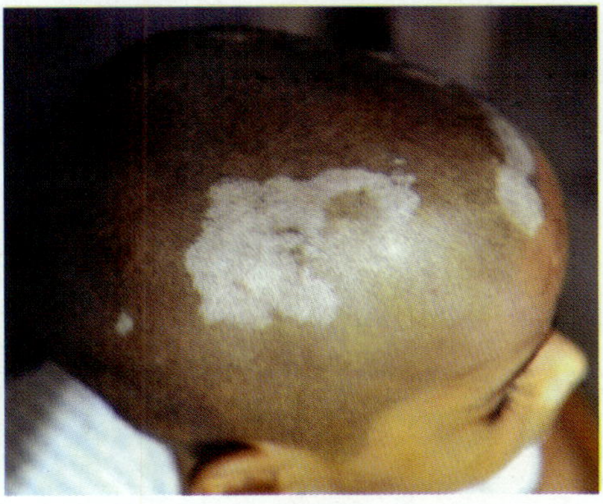

Fig. 4.9: Leucoderma–scalp child

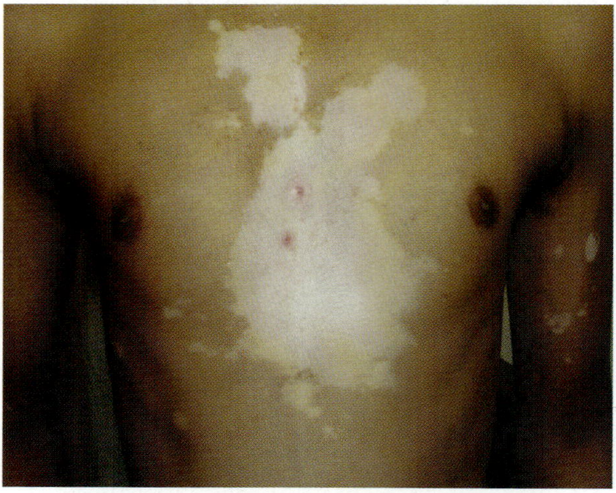

Fig. 4.10: Leucoderma–chest

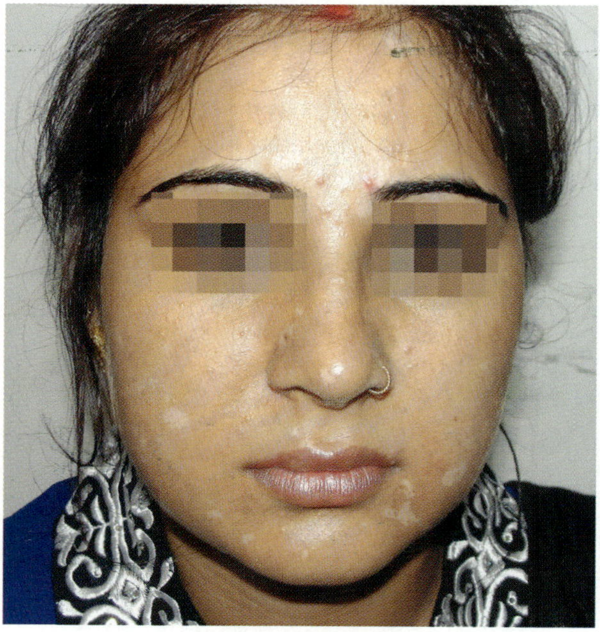

Fig. 4.11: Leucoderma–face

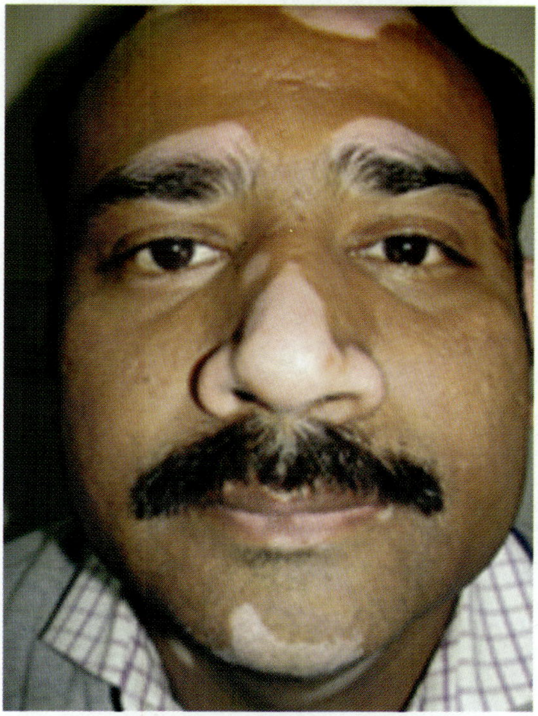

Fig. 4.12: Leucoderma–face

(arms and legs) or the trunk are the sites commonly involved. The disease may remain limited to a few lesions only or it may progress to form different patterns. In some patients, the disease remains confined to the face or peripheral parts of the extremities or both, while in others the lesions are limited to the lips, soles, toes, fingertips and mucous membrane of private parts like glans penis and vulva. The lesions may be bilaterally symmetrical or have no particular pattern of distribution and scattered randomly on any part of the body. There may be extensive involvement of the body sparing a few residual normal color areas, which are commonly located on the face or the extensor surface of the forearms.

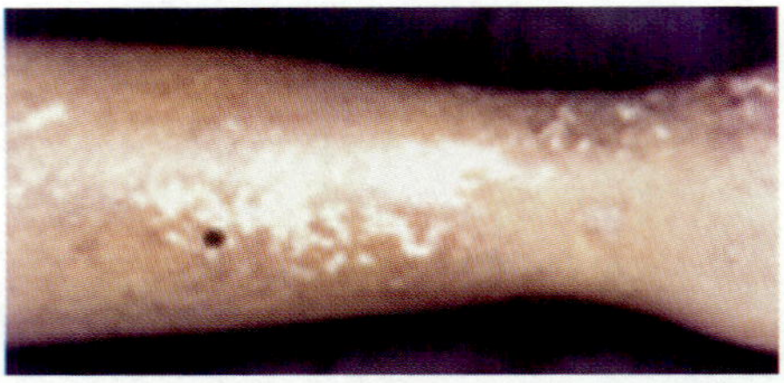

Fig. 4.13: Leucoderma leg–follicular repigmentation with treament

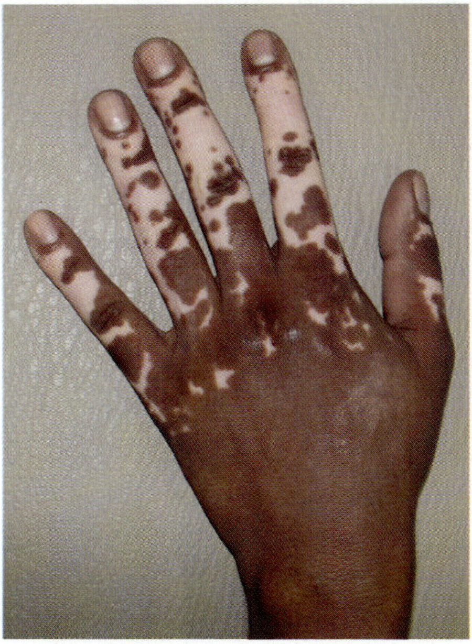

Fig. 4.14: Leucoderma–dorsum of hand

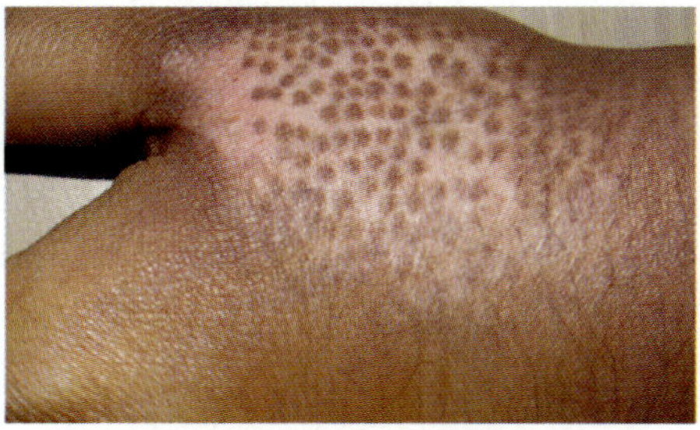

Fig. 4.15: Leucoderma hand–during treatment

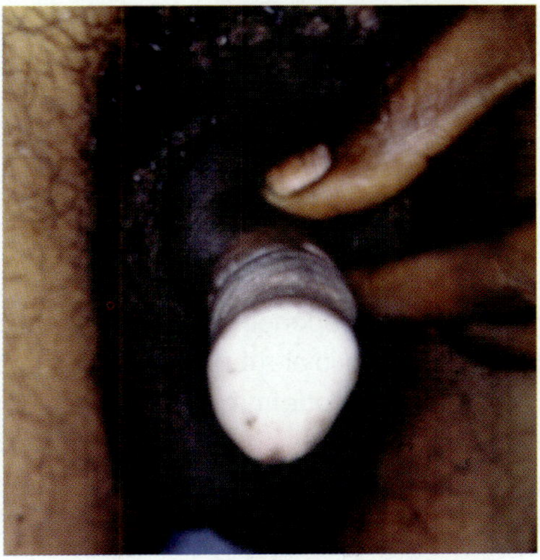

Fig. 4.22: Leucoderma–glans

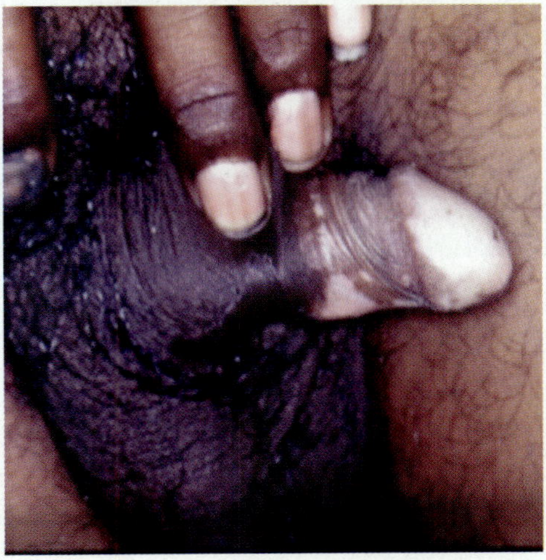

Fig. 4.23: Leucoderma–glans and shaft of penis

In some patients, the leucoderma lesions may predominantly be present on the flexural aspect. Some patients have lesions predominantly on the sun-exposed areas and these may show aggravation on exposure to the sun.

The distribution of some of the lesions may show a pattern suggestive of their relationship to their cause. Presence of lesions on the flanks corresponding to the area under the saree or the salwar string suggests the possible role of pressure.

Localization of the lesions in the 'Bindi' area of the forehead, upper part of the left breast in a right-handed lady and in the right breast in a left handed one corrosponding to area of the purse. On the dorsum of the feet corresponding to the footwear or other areas coming in contact with plastic or rubber agents suggests the role of chemicals. Such type of leucoderma does not occur in all the people using these agents, thus, susceptibility of the individual is an important factor. Some patients develop depigmentation at the sites of trauma especially the knees, elbows, malleoli and the knuckles.

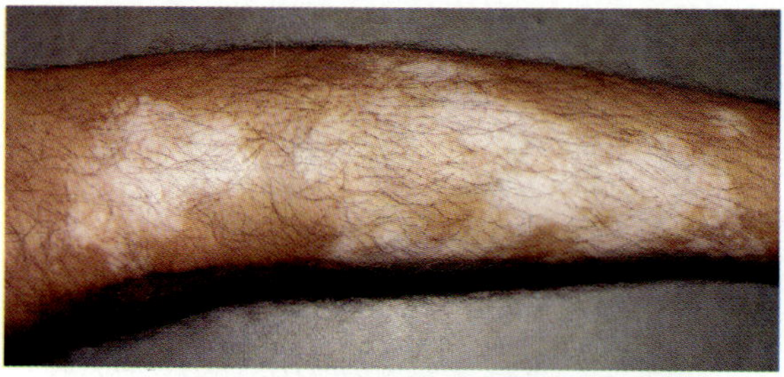

Fig. 4.24: Leucoderma–cubital fossa

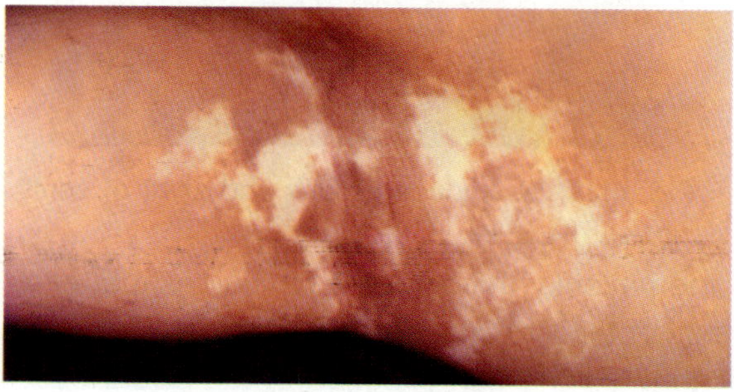

Fig. 4.25: Leucoderma–axilla

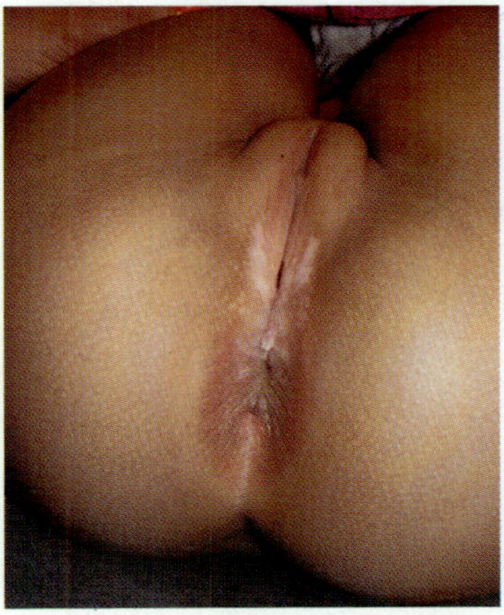

Fig. 4.26: Leucoderma–female genital

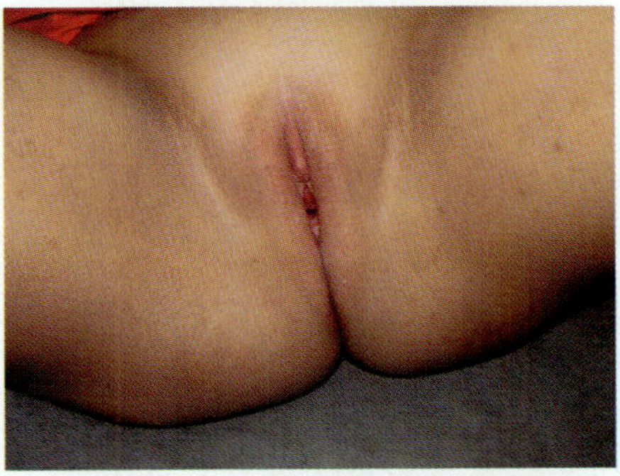

Fig. 4.27: Leucoderma–female genital

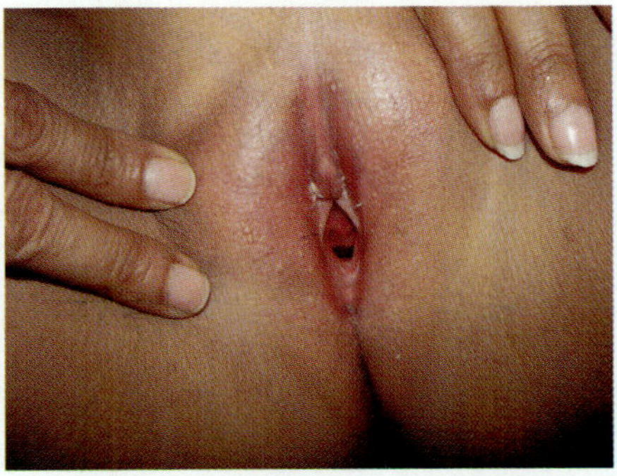

Fig. 4.28: Leucoderma–female genital after treatment

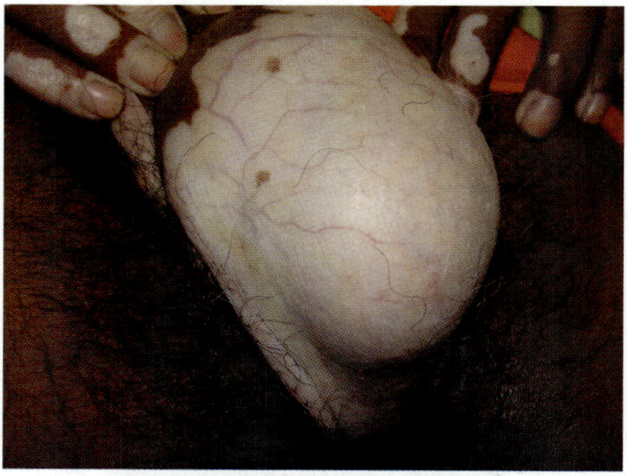

Fig. 4.29: Leucoderma–scrotum

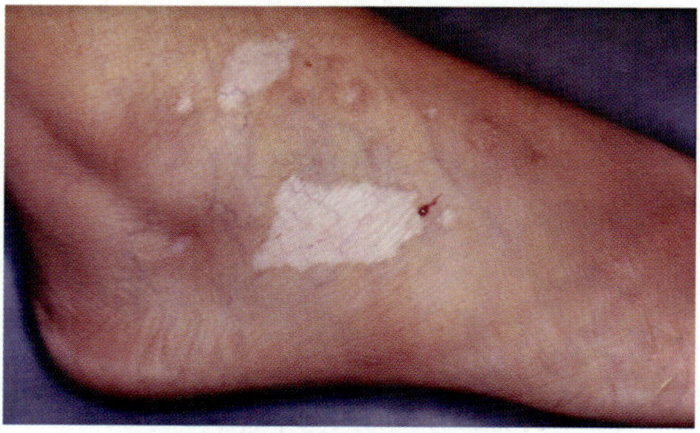

Fig. 4.30: Leucoderma–ankle

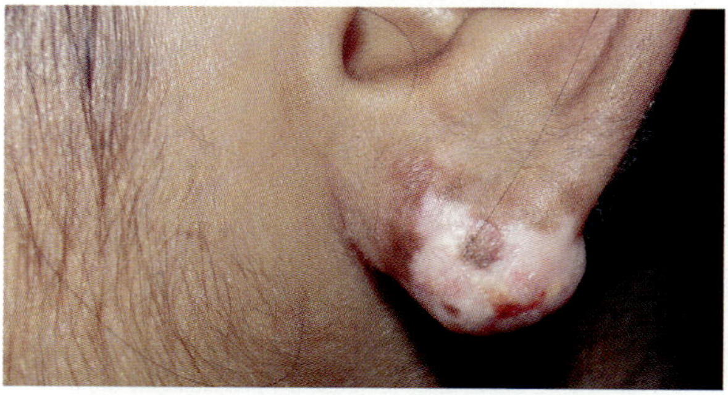

Fig. 4.31: Leucoderma ear lobule–after cryo

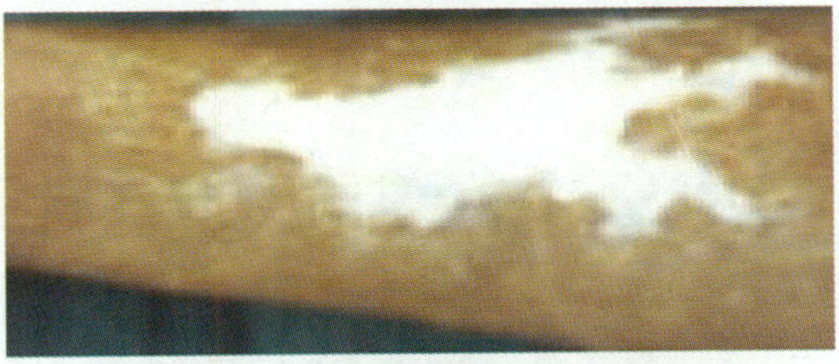

Fig. 4.32: Leucoderma–at site of burn

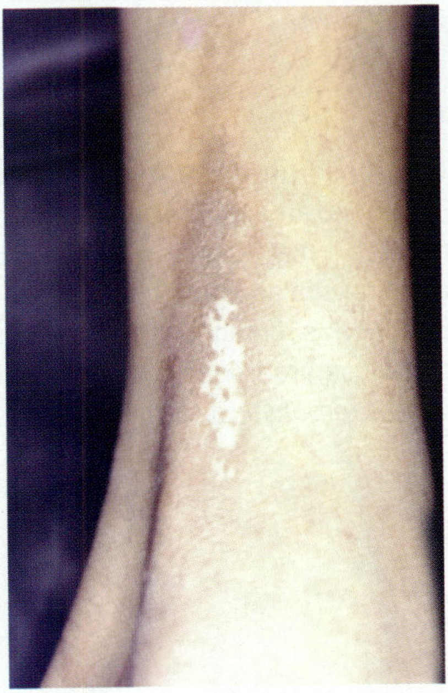

Fig. 4.33: Leucoderma–on lichen simplex chronicus

The trauma may be minor and may remain unnoticed. Such patients also have the tendency to develop depigmentation at sites of scratch marks.

Some patients, have halo naevi in association with leucoderma or occasionally just a halo naevus, or develop depigmentation in the scar(s) due to surgery, trauma or vaccination much before the onset of leucoderma.

CHAPTER

5 Diseases Confused for Leucoderma

PITYRIASIS ALBA

It occurs mainly in children and presents as asymptomatic, hypopigmented, ill-defined areas, usually on cheeks and other parts of the face. Sometimes it may also be seen on other parts of the body. Occasionally, fine scales may be present on the patch. The lesions usually disappear spontaneously after being present for a long period. Recurrences are frequent but rare after puberty. It is believed to be due to *saprophytic* bacteria called *staphylococcus.*

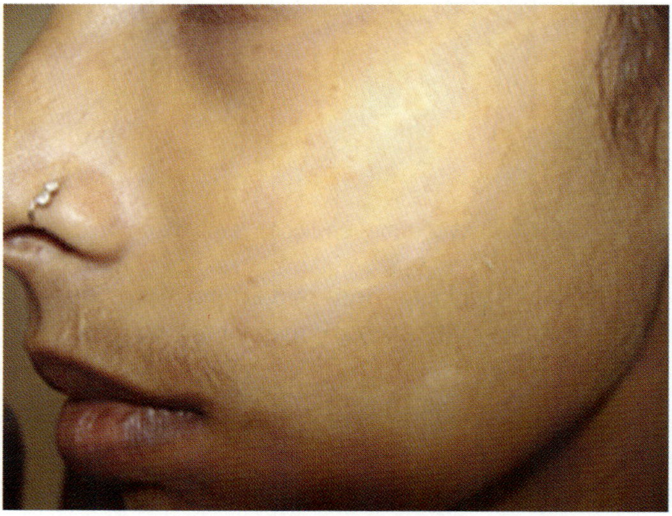

Fig. 5.1: Pityriasis alba–hypopigmented fine scaly areas on face

PITYRIASIS VERSICOLOR

It is a common fungal infection that presents as slightly scaly, hypopigmented macules mainly on upper trunk which may spread to shoulder, upper arms, lower trunk and neck. The earliest lesions are usually located around the hair follicles but may soon coalesce to involve large area. The causative organism *Malassezia furfur* can easily be demonstrated in scrapings from the lesions in 10% KOH solution.

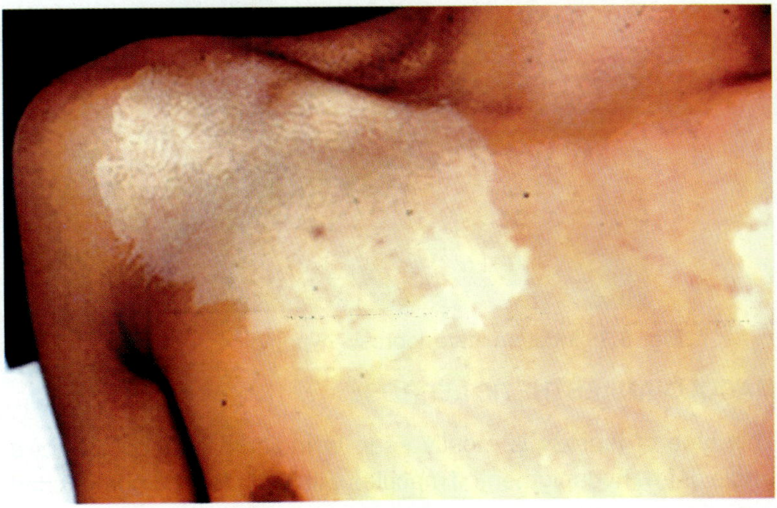

Fig. 5.2: Pityriasis versicolor–hypopigmented areas on chest

INDETERMINATE LEPROSY

It presents as asymptomatic, ill-defined, hypopigmented area(s) with doubtful loss of sensations.

Careful examination of well-stained serial sections of the skin lesion may reveal acid-fast bacilli in dermal nerve fibrils, infiltrated with lymphocytes. Many of these lesions disappear spontaneously without any treatment. Thus, the patient of indeterminate leprosy should be examined at 3 to 6 months interval to assess the progress of the disease.

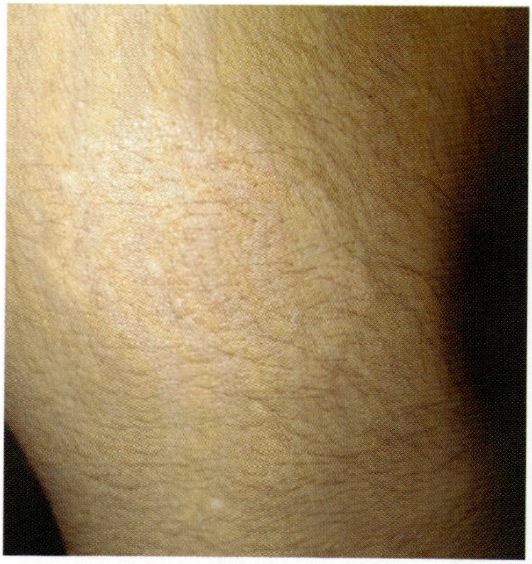

Fig. 5.3: Indeterminate leprosy–hypopigmented areas

MACULO-ANAESTHETIC LEPROSY

This type of leprosy is mostly seen in Indians and consists of a single or few hypopigmented macules with well-defined borders and loss of superficial sensations. Regional nerve may be enlarged.

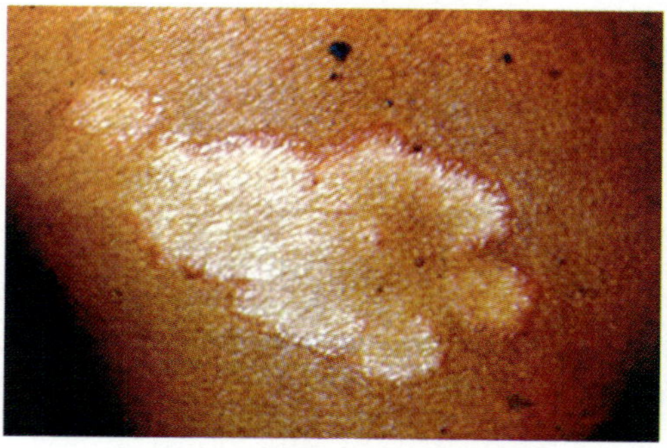

Fig. 5.4: Maculo-anaesthetic leprosy–hypopigmented areas

NAEVUS ACHROMICUS

It is also known as naevus depigmentosus and presents as asymptomatic depigmented or occasionally hypopigmented macules (areas), confined to one side of the body corresponding usually to a neural segment. The lesion of naevus achromicus is usually present at birth or appears early in life but does not spread or increase in size later on.

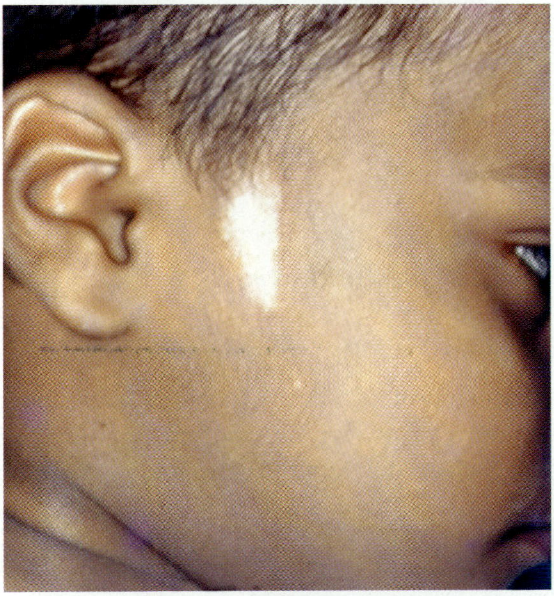

Fig. 5.5: Naevus achromicus

WHITE MACULES OF TUBEROUS SCLEROSIS

The leaf-shaped white macules of tuberous sclerosis vary from 1 to 3 cm in length and are usually seen on the trunk or limbs. It is usually present at birth or in early infancy and may be associated with other cutaneous lesions of tuberous sclerosis and mental retardation, which is usually progressive.

Depigmented lesions are static and do not increase in size or spread later in life.

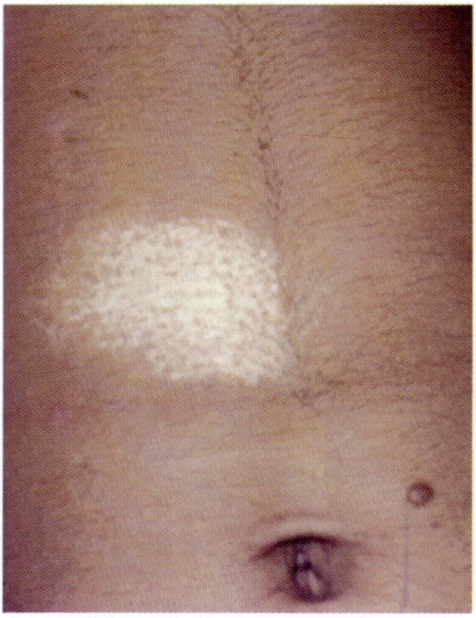

Fig. 5.6: White macules in tuberous sclerosis

POST KALA-AZAR DERMAL LEISHMANIASIS (PKDL)

In a small proportion of kala-azar patients in India, the skin rash appears 1-2 years after recovery as hypopigmented macules all over the body, especially on the trunk. The hypopigmented macules are

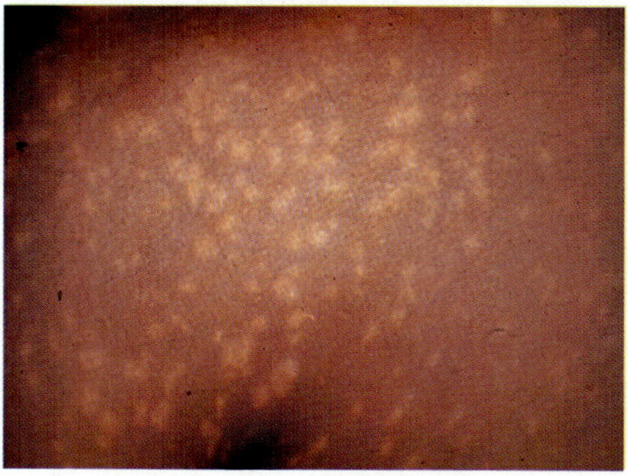

Fig. 5.7: Post kala-azar dermal leishmaniasis

progressive and seldom heal spontaneously. After a variable period, diffuse nodules may develop on these macules. Biopsy shows poorly differentiated infiltrate, with variable number of leishmania in dermal macrophages.

PITYRIASIS LICHENOIDES CHRONICA (PLC)

The lesions of both acute and chronic forms sometimes leave behind transient depigmented areas that may persist for a prolong period. Such depigmented, sometimes atrophic areas are usually seen on the trunk and may be associated with classical small, firm, lichenoid 3-10 mm size papules with mica like adherent scales on the top.

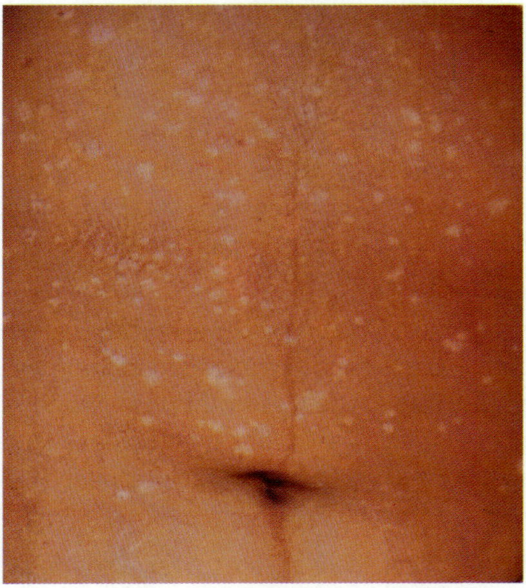

Fig. 5.8: Pityriasis lichenoides chronica–depigmented macules

CHAPTER

6 Natural Course of Leucoderma

The natural course of leucoderma varies in different individuals. In some individuals, spontaneous repigmentation of some lesions has been observed and occasionally in some, the disease may clear completely even without any treatment. Most of the time the disease worsens with a variable speed.

In some cases the lesion(s) may increase in size to a limited extent, become stationary and then remain the same. Alternatively, the lesion(s) may continue to increase in size along with appearance of new ones on other areas.

The rate at which the lesions increase in size or the new lesions appear can vary from a slow and steady increase over several years to a very rapid spread, tending to involve almost the entire skin within a few months. It is also not necessary that the disease will continue to spread progressively. The lesions may increase for some time, become stationary and remain so for prolong periods. After which they may progress rapidly.

Even with treatment, there are a lot of variations depending upon a variety of factors. The repigmentation in the lesions generally starts in the perifollicular areas, though occasionally the repigmentation may occur from the periphery or the entire lesion may regain the original normal color. Different lesions may behave/respond in a different manner, even in the same patient. The quality of repigmentation may also vary. It may exactly match the color of the normal skin or it may be slightly fainter or hyperpigmented. Certain areas show a better response as compared to others. Elbows, forearms, knees, legs, some parts of the face such as the forehead, the cheeks and the chin generally show better result than the palms, soles, finger-tips, toe-tips, malleolar areas, eyelids, retro-auricular areas, flanks, areola of the nipples and the mucosal areas. In an individual patient however, these observations may not be correct and there may be any pattern of repigmentation. Thus, it is not possible to predict the future course of the disease in a particular patient.

CHAPTER

7

Treatment of Leucoderma

Leucoderma is generally considered to be an incurable disease, but this is actually not true. Many patients are impatient and tend to judge the results of treatment earlier than expected. The main approach for treatment of this disease till date has been to induce repigmentation in the white areas, while almost no efforts has been made to control the disease process. To achieve the best results, therefore, it is essential that the disease is treated in all its aspects. Thus the treatment of leucoderma should include:

1. Removing the causative/precipitating factor(s), wherever applicable.
2. Arresting the activity of the disease, if it is still active.
3. Stimulating re-pigmentation in the existing lesions; and
4. Surgical intervention in areas that do not repigment with drugs.

REMOVAL OF THE CAUSATIVE/PRECIPITATING FACTOR(S)

Since some cases of leucoderma are caused/precipitated by contact with rubber or plastic articles and possibly inhalation or ingestion of the relevant chemicals, such patients should be informed about the causative agents and advised to avoid further contact/exposure to these materials.

In cases where leucoderma is caused by pressure of the petticoat string or other articles of wearing apparel, the patient should be advised to loosen the pressure or interpose multiple layers of a handkerchief or a similar thick cotton cloth between the skin and the tight string. This would redistribute the pressure to a wider area and prevent further damage.

Individuals having leucoderma lesions located at trauma prone sites should be instructed to wear clothes which protect the areas. In patient having halo naevus, surgical removal of the mole tends to reverse the process.

It is however, not necessary to take all of these precautions in each leucoderma patient because not all the factors are operative in every patient. The approach would therefore be to ascertain if a particular factor is responsible in a particular patient and then only one should take appropriate measure to remove the effect of the causative factor in that patient.

CONTROLLING THE ACTIVITY OF LEUCODERMA

For controlling the activity of leucoderma it is essential to obtain an accurate history of the patient, right from the time of onset of the disease. The response to the treatment(s) taken by the patient so far should also be recorded to know the behavior of the disease in the patient. It is also necessary to record the state of activity of the disease at the time of presentation and in the recent past. It is essential that the history should be accurate so that the patient does not misguide you because of ignorance. Photographic records are important for objective evaluation.

Close-up life size photographs of all the lesions at the time of starting the treatment are very helpful, during subsequent follow-up evaluation. These photographs are useful to judge whether the lesions have indeed become static, and if there is any other lesion which has appeared during this period. Repigmentation or disappearance of lesions is also obvious in the photographic records. The photographs are repeated whenever there is adequate change in the size of the lesion(s).

For controlling the activity of the disease, following two schedules are quite effective:

LEVAMISOLE PULSES

Levamisole has been used for leucoderma as an immuno-modulator (correction of immunity). It is given in a dose of 150 mg orally on two consecutive days per week. But the dose has to be reduced to 100 mg for children between 6 - 12 years and 50 mg if the child is less than six years of age. The tablet can be taken at any time of the day on any two consecutive days of the week but taking the tablets at night with meals seems to be most convenient.

With this treatment, the progression of the disease gets arrested in 80 to 90% of the cases within two to four months.

Approximately half the patients start developing spontaneous repigmentation of the lesions even without any additional treatment. The treatment is continued till either all the lesions disappear or there is no further repigmentation in any of the lesions.

This is useful for patients having slowly progressive (mildly active) disease. If the patient does not show complete control of the disease activity, he/she is shifted to another treatment.

Most of the patients tolerate levamisole very well, though nausea or a vague feeling of discomfort for a variable duration after taking the drug is quite common.

In most cases, the symptoms are mild and can be ignored or treated with appropriate drugs. The other side effects with levamisole include an altered sensation of taste, insomnia, joint pains and arthritis. It is, however, necessary to confirm in each case that these side effects occur only on taking the drug, disappear when the medicine is stopped and there is recurrence on re-administration of the drug.

There is only a small percentage of patients who get severe side effects from levamisole, which necessitates interruption of the treatment.

Patients, who develop severe side effects, or those whose disease activity cannot be controlled with levamisole or who have a rapid-spreading disease, can be treated with alternative methods of treatment.

CORTICOSTEROID PULSES

Corticosteroids given systemically are very effective in controlling the activity of the disease in almost all the cases, provided one uses an adequate dose. Generally 20 to 30 mg prednisolone a day or an equivalent dose (2 to 3 mg) of betamethasone or dexamethasone is sufficient. This dose however, used over a prolong period can lead to a variety of side effects, such as obesity, swollen face, diabetes mellitus, hypertension, peptic ulcer, acne, striae atrophicans, hirsutism, osteoporosis, etc. Although most of these side effects are reversible on stopping the treatment, most patients do not like these side effects especially when the disease itself is only a cosmetic problem. Betamethasone or dexamethasone 5 mg as a single oral dose on two consecutive days per week is capable of producing the therapeutic effect without producing significant side effects.

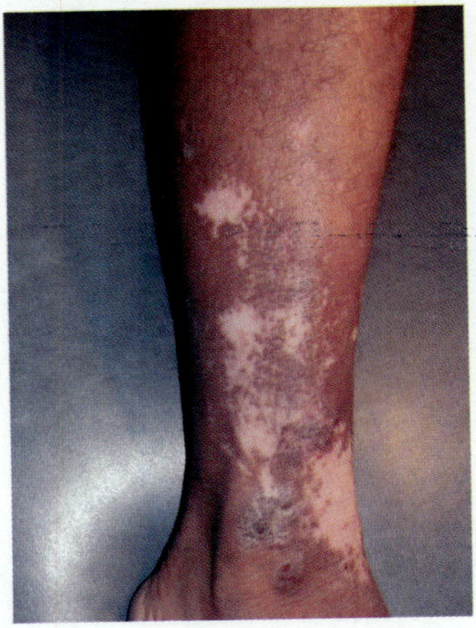

Fig. 7.1: Leucoderma–leg on treatment

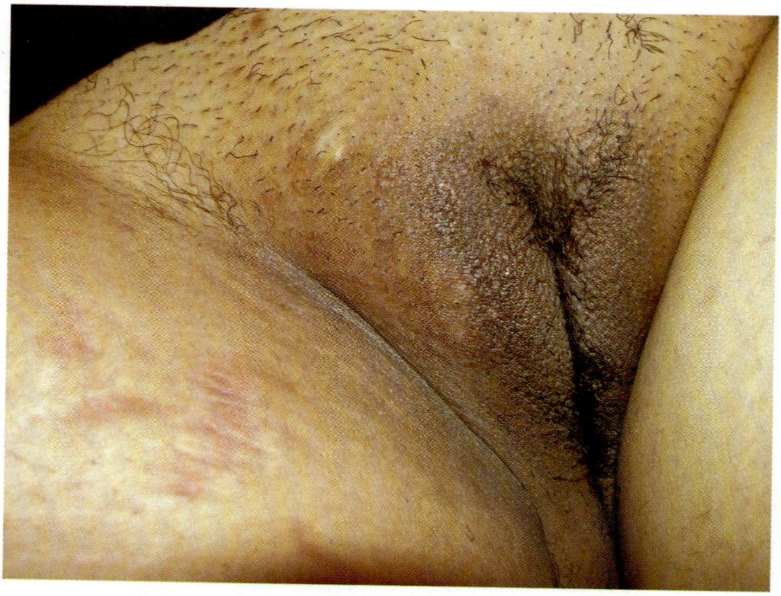

Fig. 7.2: Leucoderma–mons pubis on treatment

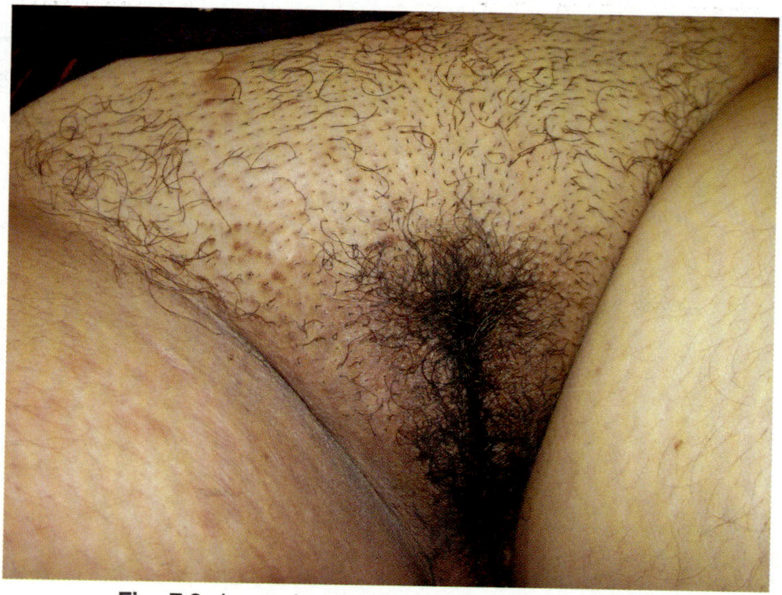

Fig. 7.3: Leucoderma–almost treated mons pubis

All the tablets should be taken together after breakfast. For children, this dose can be calculated on the basis of body weight, using 0.5 mg betamethasone for every 5 kg of body weight.

Patients having diabetes mellitus, hypertension, peptic ulcer or any other disease can also be given this treatment, but treatment for underlying disease will have to be continued. Pregnant women preferably should not be given this treatment.

Within one to two months of starting the treatment, progression of the disease gets arrested in about 90 percent of the patients. Several patients notice spontaneous repigmentation of the existing lesions. The rate and extent of repigmentation varies in different patients; some patients show complete or almost complete repigmentation of all the lesions, while some others may not obtain any significant repigmentation. The treatment has to be continued as long as any one of the lesions is showing repigmentation or till complete repigmentation of all the lesions. After achieving complete/ maximal repigmentation, the dose of corticosteroids should be gradually reduced stepwise over a period of 6-8 months.

With this, there have been no side effects commonly observed with systemic corticosteroids, although, the patient may experience a transient increase in appetite, or puffiness of the face on the day of taking the drug, and temporary lethargy or weakness one or two days after the pulse. These side effects occur only in an occasional patient, and can be managed with symptomatic treatment. This regimen of treatment is equally safe for older individuals and children. The children continue to gain their height and weight as per normal expectations. This treatment can be continued even for a few years, if the patient is showing an adequate response.

In case the progression of the disease is not completely arrested with 5 mg betamethasone on two consecutive days per week, the optimum result can be achieved by increasing the dose to 7.5 mg on two consecutive days per week, for a period of six to nine months. With this dose however, the patient is likely to have an increase in the body weight and other minor side effects of corticosteroids. These side effects however, disappear when this phase of treatment is over and the dose is reduced to 5 mg on two consecutive days per week. The gain in body weight can also be minimized by adjusting the food intake by the patient. The patient should be advised to take more of vegetables and pulses and reduce the intake of cereals and fat as far as possible, during this period.

Alternatively, patients who do not obtain adequate control of the disease with standard oral pulse therapy can be supplemented with 50 mg cyclophosphamide taken orally on all days of the week. This low dose of cyclophosphamide is also devoid of any side effects known to occur with cyclophosphamide and can even be continued for several years, if necessary. For children, however, cyclophosphamide should be avoided.

STIMULATING PIGMENTATION IN EXISTING LESIONS

Once the activity of the disease has been effectively controlled and the influence of the precipitating factors removed, many patients start developing repigmentation in their lesions even without any other additional treatment. This repigmentation, however, does not occur in all the patients and in all the lesions even in the same patient.

Sunlight acts as a natural stimulant of pigmentation. Therefore, the lesions situated on the sun-exposed areas tend to repigment earlier. Rarely, however, patients have been encountered where the leucoderma lesions are located entirely or predominantly on the sun-exposed areas and show aggravation whenever the patient is excessively exposed to sunlight. It would be necessary to identify such cases at the earliest, prevent exposure to sunlight as far as possible and treat them with oral or local corticosteroids.

Psoralens (a drug given to stimulate pigmentation in presence of sunlight) in such patients should be avoided.

Patients who do not show a tendency for spontaneous repigmentation within four to six months of starting the treatment, or those where it is necessary to obtain repigmentation at a faster rate, should be given additional treatment to stimulate pigmentation. This can be done in a variety of ways as follow.

TOPICAL CORTICOSTEROIDS

Corticosteroid ointments applied and massage on leucoderma lesions have been observed to lead to repigmentation in 70 to 80 percent of the patients. It is sufficient to apply the ointment once a day at any convenient time, but it is necessary to massage the ointment adequately into the lesion. Moderate to high potency corticosteroids such as betamethasone dipropionate, mometasone, fluticasone, beclomethasone dipropionate, and fluocinolone acetonide have been found useful for this purpose. Low potency topical corticosteroids, however, may not be effective. Contrary to experience quoted in

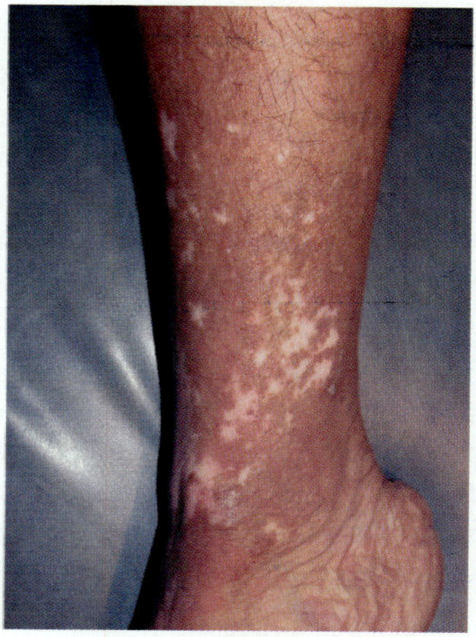

Fig. 7.4: Leucoderma leg–on treatment

literature, topical application of these high potency corticosteroids do not produce side effects such as atrophy, telangiectasia, acne and hirsutism in Indians. In a small percentage of patients, where these side effects are observed, these changes are reversible on interrupting the treatment, if detected early. Clobetasol propionate ointment has been found to be more effective, but the incidence of local side effects is very high, even among Indians. In addition, this drug produces a diffuse area of hypopigmentation around the lesion, leading to a false apprehension that the leucoderma lesion has increased in size. Even though this hypopigmentation is reversible on stopping the treatment.

PUVA/PUVASOL

There is a group of chemical substances, called 'furocoumarins', produced by a plant, which induce pigmentation of the skin if contact with the plant is followed by exposure to sunlight. Without exposure to sunlight, these compounds do not produce pigmentation.

These chemical compounds are called 'photosensitizers'. Two such products derived from the plant, *Psoralea corylifolia* in India and *Ammi majus* in Egypt, have been used since ancient times for the treatment of leucoderma. Psoralea corylifolia is commonly known as Babchi and has been used in Ayurveda in the form of seeds, extracts or concoctions for topical as well as oral administration. Psoralens are present in the leaves, fruits, seeds, roots and rhizomes of the plants.

Subsequently, the active ingredients of these plants have been identified and synthesized at a commercial scale for therapeutic purposes. These compounds are collectively known as 'psoralens'. Psoralens at present are considered to be the most effective and dependable therapeutic agent for the treatment of leucoderma. Four types of psoralens are in common use which include:

1. The parent compound, psoralen.
2. 3, 5, 8-trimethyl psoralen (TMP).

3. 8-methoxy psoralen (8-MOP); and

4. 5-methoxypsoralen (5-MOP).

All these compounds are very potent in sensitizing the skin to UVA (320-400 nm) spectrum of ultraviolet (UV) radiation. They are almost equally effective and can be used interchangeably, except that some are relatively more toxic and have the tendency to produce more erythema and blistering than others. 5-MOP has been reported to produce the minimum side effects. These drugs can be used topically as well as orally, but the skin should be exposed to UVA light within a specific time after the use of the drug.

Use of psoralens followed by exposure to UVA radiations from an artificial source of light, is called 'PUVA', while the use of sunlight as the source of UVA radiations following psoralens, is called 'PUVASOL'. The dose of psoralens for oral therapy consists of 0.3 to 0.6 mg/kg body weight for 8-MOP, 0.5 to 0.8 mg/kg for trimethyl psoralen, and 0.6 to 1.2 mg/kg for 5-MOP. This dosage can be rounded off to 20 to 40 mg for an average adult. The dose for children should be reduced proportionately, but children below twelve years of age should not be treated with oral psoralens. It takes two hours after oral intake for the drug to attain maximum concentration in the skin and this level is generally maintained for another two hours. It is therefore, best to take the drug as a single oral dose and to expose the lesions to UVA radiations for two to four hours after oral administration of the drug. When using artificial source of light (PUVA), the time of ingestion of the drug and exposure to the UVA can be fixed according to the convenience of the patient. However when using PUVASOL which is a cheaper method of treatment, specially in a country where plenty of sunlight is available, it is best to expose to sunlight at noon, between 12.00 - 2.00 p.m. Because the intensity of UVA is maximum during this period. It would, thus, be better to take the drug at 10.00 a.m. and expose the lesions to sunlight between 12.00 - 2.00 p.m.

The duration of exposure to UVA has to be adjusted depending on several factors. The reactivity of the skin to UVA varies from individual to individual and also in different regions of the body. When using sunlight as the source of UVA, the intensity of the light reaching the surface of earth varies from place to place and from day to day and also whether the atmosphere is clear, dusty or cloudy.

An optimum exposure to UVA should be able to induce pigmentation in the skin lesions without producing any other effect. Most patients in addition tend to develop a mild erythema, which can be ignored. An over exposure, however, can lead to intense erythema, scaling and even blistering along with burning sensation and pain. It is therefore, preferable to start with short duration of exposure and progressively increase the duration till the lesions start showing repigmentation. In case the patient develops severe erythema and scaling, the duration of exposure should be reduced and in case of blistering, the treatment should be stopped temporarily till the blisters heal. Local and/or systemic corticosteroids in an appropriate dose can be used to control the unwanted reaction(s). After the reaction has subsided, treatment with PUVA/PUVASOL can be restarted, using a shorter duration of UVA exposure.

It is customary to start with 10-15 minutes of exposure to sunlight and progressively increase it to a maximum of 30 minutes. While using PUVA, the dosage is calculated in terms of joules/cm^2. In case vitiligo is limited to a few lesions only, one can use topical PUVA/PUVASOL, which consists of applying psoralens on the lesions locally, followed by exposure to the UVA lamp or sunlight.

The side effects to oral psoralens include nausea, vomiting, headache and dizziness. These symptoms have been recorded in only a small percentage of patients and are usually mild. The symptoms can either be ignored or the patient may be given concomitant adjuvant treatment to control the symptoms. It has also been recorded that psoralens may damage the liver in a few cases. For this reason it is advisable to do liver function tests during the first six months of treatment to ensure that the liver is not being affected.

PUVA therapy has also been reported to lead to some autoimmune disorders and malignancies if used for very prolong periods. Occasionally, sudden exacerbations of vitiligo have been seen on using PUVA/PUVASOL. In such cases, this treatment should be avoided. It should also be avoided in patients having skin diseases caused by sunlight or when the vitiligo lesions are almost exclusively located on the sun-exposed areas of the body. PUVA is also reported to cause cataract. Patients on oral psoralens are therefore, recommended either to wear sunglasses during the day to protect their eyes, or use PUVA therapy in the evening so that a major proportion of the psoralen gets excreted during the night. Some dermatologists advise the use of topical emollient on the adjoining normal skin before exposure to UVA to prevent hyperpigmentation in these areas. In most cases, this is not needed.

The major limitation of PUVA therapy is the cumbersome nature of the entire procedure. Most patients find it difficult to expose their skin lesions to UVA at the appropriate time of day because they may be busy in their routine work at the time when they are expected to expose to UVA. Women often find it difficult to expose their skin to sunlight if the lesions are located on their private parts.It is also costly and inconvenient to visit the PUVA clinics frequently for prolong period.

On the days when it is not possible to expose to UVA during the stipulated period, because of occupational or other commitments or if there is no sunlight at the appropriate time because of cloudy weather, the patient can be asked to expose to UVA at the earliest possible, but increase the duration of exposure.

Generally, the PUVA/PUVASOL therapy is given 2-3 times a week and should be continued as long as the lesions are getting repigmented. If there is no repigmentation in any of the lesions in spite of adequate and proper treatment for 6 months, the treatment may be considered to have failed. PUVA/PUVASOL therapy should not be used in children below 12 years of age, pregnancy, lactation, photosensitive skin diseases, melanoma or patients who have received treatment with arsenic or ionising radiation or those with severe heart, kidney or liver disease. Care is also necessary if the patient is concomitantly receiving treatment with photosensitizing drugs such as sulphonamides, hypoglycemic agents, dimethylchlortetracycline, griseofulvin or phenothiazines. The patient must wear UV-opaque goggles during the UVA exposure and UVA-protective glasses for at least 12 hours after exposure to prevent the development of cataract and also sun-protective clothing for at least 8 hours after the oral dose. Some skin specialists therefore prefer to give PUVA therapy in the evening so that the psoralen gets excreted during the night and thus there is no need for protection from natural sunlight.

Repigmentation following PUVA/PUVASOL in majority of the cases, starts around the areas of hair follicles. Lesions on the face and neck and those which are of recent origin respond better especially if the disease is limited to a few areas only, while the skin areas such as the palms and soles, dorsal aspects of the fingers and toes, and mucosal areas which do not have hair follicles, or if the hair follicles have also lost their melanocytes (leucotrichia), do not repigment easily. In some cases however, the lesion regains its pigmentation by migration of the pigmented border from the adjoining normal skin or the entire skin may get repigmented because there were possibly some viable melanocytes in the lesion itself. The success of the treatment depends upon whether there are enough melanocytes present in the hair follicles/basal cell layer of the lesion or the adjoining skin, which can be stimulated to migrate into the lesion and whether the procedure has been carried out effectively. Inadequate dosage, insufficient exposure to UVA, irregularities in taking the treatment, expecting the results too early and impatience on the part of the patient can all contribute to the failure of the treatment. Repigmentation following PUVA/PUVASOL is generally darker than the normal skin color of the patient and many patients often feel embarrassed by this hyperpigmentation. With time however, the color tends to reduce and match the normal complexion. 5-methoxypsoralen (5-MOP) is another naturally occurring psoralen,

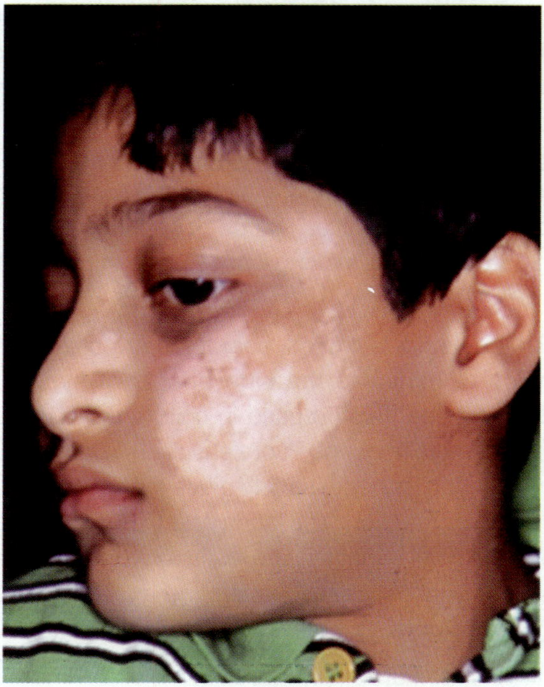

Fig. 7.5: Leucoderma face–repigmentation with treatment

which is as effective as 8-MOP but has fewer and less frequent side effects. In equivalent doses it does not lead to phototoxicity or nausea. It can therefore be used in a higher dose (0.6-1.2 mg/kg body weight) and thus it has been claimed to produce a better therapeutic effect.

4,5,8-trimethyl psoralen (TMP) is a synthetic derivative of methoxypsoralen, but it is poorly absorbed from the gastro-intestinal tract. It is thus considered to be less effective than 8-MOP. It is chiefly recommended for local application and skin exposure (photo-chemotherapy), but several skin specialists use it for systemic photochemotherapy also. The recommended dose for oral therapy is 0.8-1.2 mg/kg body weight.

Recently, an ultramicronized form of 8-MOP has been used for the treatment of leucoderma. The smaller size of the particles helps to increase the absorption of the drug from the gastro-intestinal tract and thus reduce the incidence of side effects. A dose of 0.25 mg/kg body weight given to leucoderma patients resulted in 75-100% repigmentation in patients, and a higher dose of 0.5 mg/kg body weight produce better results. The peak concentration of the drug reached in 35-55 minutes making it possible to expose to UVA at an earlier time.

When the disease is limited, psoralens are used locally. Local therapy helps to minimize the side effects of systemic PUVA/ PUVASOL and it can also be used in children. But the phototoxic reactions are far more frequent. Psoralens are available as 0.1- 0.75% creams or lotion but it is necessary to dilute them 10-20 times further to avoid phototoxic reaction. The lotion/cream is applied on the white areas and after 15-30 minutes the area is exposed to either sunlight for 1-5 minutes or UVA lamp. The starting dose of UVA for Indian skin is 0.25 J/cm^2 or even less.

This dose is then gradually increased to a maximum of 2 J/cm^2 depending upon the tolerance or the therapeutic effect, in the same manner as for oral PUVA/PUVASOL.

However, it must be re-emphasized that the dose of sunlight/ UVA has to be increased gradually and carefully to avoid phototoxic reaction, which are far more frequent with topical PUVA/ PUVASOL. After exposure to sunlight/UVA, it is necessary to protect the area from sunlight otherwise inadvertent exposure to sunlight even for a very brief period is likely to induce severe phototoxic reactions.

NARROW BAND UVB

Narrow Band UVB with a spectrum of 311nm has also been found to be useful in the treatment of leucoderma. It has been found to be the most effective treatment for widespread leucoderma. Treatment is given 2-3 times every week. It should not be given on two consecutive days.

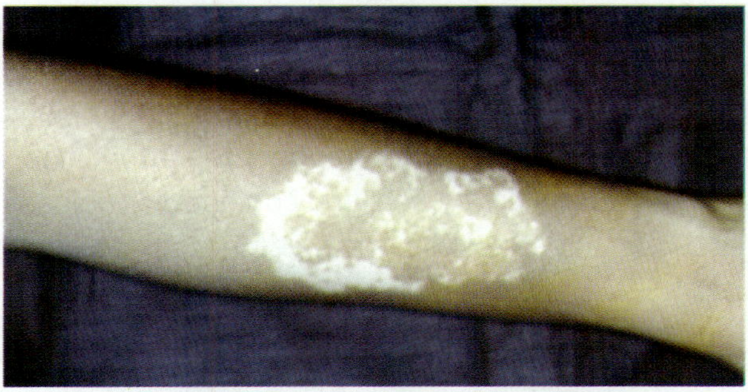

Fig. 7.6: Leucoderma leg–repigmentation with treatment

It is effective even when given alone. Immediate problem with narrow band UVB are itching and dryness which are treated with moisturizing cream. Advantage of NB UVB include no need to use sunscreen to protect from sunlight, can be used in children, pregnant and breastfeeding women and in individuals with liver and kidney diseases.

PUVB

It is like PUVA therapy. In this, patients are given psoralen 2 hours before exposure to light. Here the light used is UVB in place of UVA. It is equally effective as of PUVA therapy.

308 NM EXCIMER LASER

Narrow Band UVB with a spectrum of 308 nm has produced repigmentation when used twice weekly for a month. It has advantage over narrow band UVB, by selectively treating single leucodermic patch and sparing the unaffected areas, thus achieving improvement rapidly. Pigmentation is stable in patients treated with it.

PLACENTAL EXTRACT

It was used for the first time by an Indian skin specialist as intramuscular injections in cases of leucoderma and he observed pigmentation of the leucoderma lesions. More recently, a Cuban skin specialist has used it topically followed by exposure to infra-red rays and observed repigmentation of the leucoderma lesions. Human placenta contains a variety of components that include tyrosine, copper, pantothenic acid, cortisol and corticotropin-releasing factor which have very potent biological activities in relation to the formation of melanin.

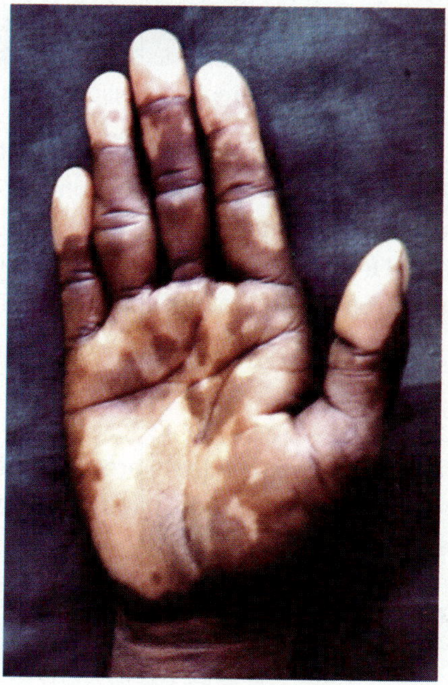

Fig. 7.7: Leucoderma palm–do not repigment easily

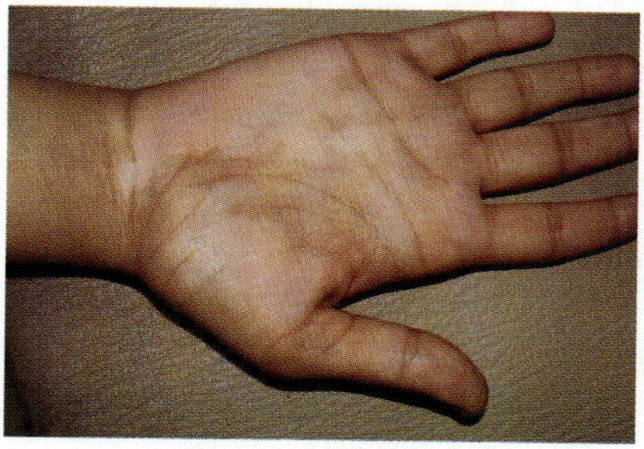

Fig. 7.8: Leucoderma palm–do not repigment easily

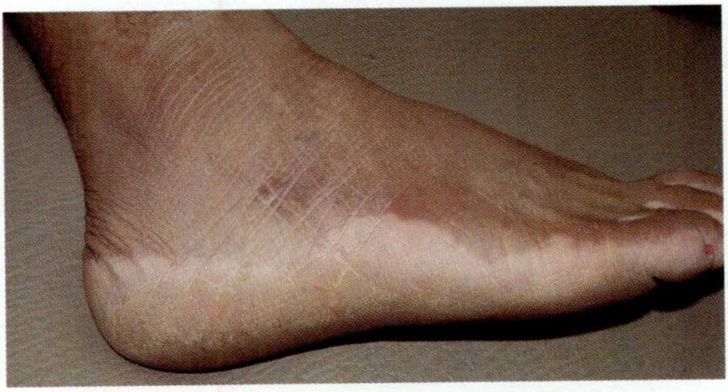

Fig. 7.9: Leucoderma side of sole–repigment poorly

However, the exact component(s) present in placental extract responsible for repigmentation is not known and the rationale for using infra-red rays is also not known. Some skin specialists have found good results even on exposure to UVA lamp or sunlight. This drug does not produce local erythema or blistering or any systemic side effects. Intramuscular injections of placental extracts do not require exposure to infra-red or UVA light by the patients. The injections are repeated at intervals of 1-7 days. The main drawback of this treatment is that the injections have to be continued for prolong periods. Placental extract has also been used intralesionally. The intralesional injections are repeated at weekly or fortnightly intervals and the repigmentation is visible within a few months. The treatment is continued till either there is repigmentation of all the lesions or there is no further repigmentation in any of the lesions for a period of at least six months.

TACROLIMUS AND PIMECROLIMUS

A topical immuno-modulator/immuno-suppressive agent, has been found producing repigmentation of leucoderma lesions when used as 0.03-0.1% ointment locally twice daily for more than 3 months.

CALCIPROTRIENE

Due to its suppressive action of the immune response, and/or its ability for inhibiting the accumulation of toxic intermediates of melanin breakdown, it starts improving the leucoderma lesions in 4-21 weeks after starting application.

KHELLIN

Khellin is isolated from the seeds of *Ammivisnaga* found in the eastern Mediterranean region. Like psoralens, it also has a photosensitizing effect. Dose of khellin is 100 mg orally daily followed by sun exposure 45 minutes later for 15 minutes. It has been observed to produce moderate to good repigmentation in 40-50% of the cases. A 2% topical solution of khellin applied on the affected areas followed by UVA exposure 1 hour later has been found to be mildly effective. The side effect include nausea, dizziness and mild elevation of liver enzymes.

PHENYLALANINE

Phenylalanine, a part of our daily diet, has also been found useful in leucoderma when used in doses of 50-100 mg/kg/day followed by exposure to UVA after one hour. No significant side effect has been observed. It is also reported to stabilize the disease process because of its ability to inhibit the synthesis of antibodies. It has also been used as a 10% topical application followed by UVA exposure after 20 minutes. It is reported to be safe and can be used in children also.

CYCLOPHOSPHAMIDE

The basis of using cyclophosphamide, an immuno-suppressive drug in leucoderma is that leucoderma is an auto-immune disease. It has been used in a dose of 50 mg twice a day and found to produce satisfactory repigmentation. It has also been used as an adjuvant with oral corticosteroids pulse therapy, 50 mg daily with very good result. The side effects observed with this dose is almost none.

TOPICAL FLUOROURACIL

This drug causes increased pigmentation of the skin when used locally or systemically. In leucoderma it is used as 5% cream for local application under occlusion after abrading the white areas. It often produces a darker pigmentation than the surrounding normal skin. It is not useful in segmental vitiligo, and sometimes the pigment disappeared after stopping the treatment.

CLOFAZIMINE

Clofazimine, a dye and an anti-leprosy drug, as a rule produces hyperpigmentation. This drug was therefore tried in the doses of 100-300 mg per day in leucoderma but the results were variable. The pigment invariably disappears after the treatment is stopped.

PSEUDO-CATALASE

A topical preparation, containing pseudo-catalase and calcium chloride applied twice a day followed by total body exposure to suberythema dose of UVB after one hour, twice a week has been observed to arrest the activity of the disease as well as produce pigmentation in the white spots.

BASIC FIBROBLAST GROWTH FACTOR (BFGF) DERIVED PEPTIDE

Topical application has been found producing repigmentation in leucoderma. It is believed to stimulate the regrowth of melanocytes in the hair roots of leucoderma lesions and the melanocytes in the skin surrounding the leucoderma patch.

OTHER DRUGS

Apart from the drugs described above, there are several other drugs which have been used by various workers to induce pigmentation in leucoderma lesions like levodopa, thiambutosine, topical tar, mechlorethamine, topical minoxidil, azathioprine, dapsone, intralesional ACTH and ludermol oil. They have been used in a few cases but their efficacy in larger group of patients has not been evaluated.

CHAPTER

8 Assessment of effects of Treatment

Response to the treatment is slow in leucoderma. Pigmentation in the lesions usually start around the hair-roots, thus, the lesions in hairy areas show early and quick response with treatment. The melanocytes present in hair follicles start dividing and migrating into the depigmented skin, leading to pigmentation around the hair follicles

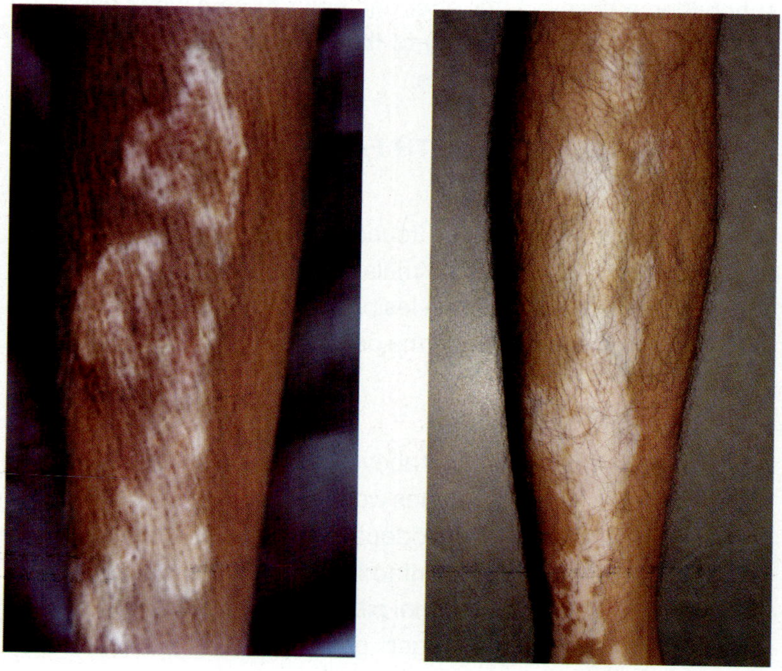

Fig. 8.1: Leucoderma leg–follicular repigmentation with treatment

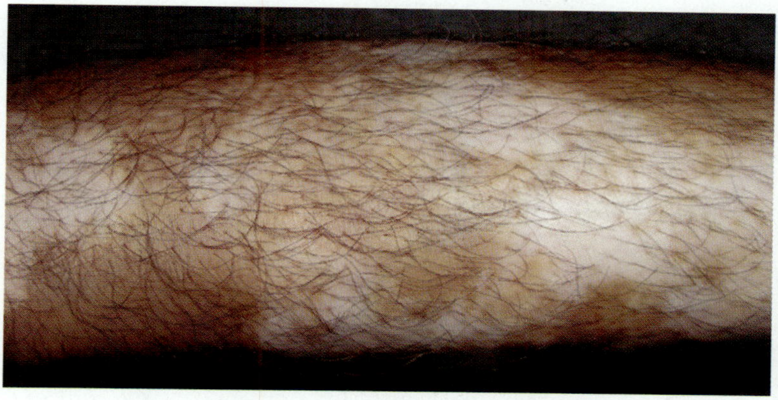

Fig. 8.2: Leucoderma leg–repigmentation with treatment

(roots). The pigmented areas gradually increase in size and merge with each other, leading to the repigmentation of the entire lesion. As a general rule, therefore, the skin areas bearing hair follicles repigment earlier and faster than non-hairy areas of the skin like palms and soles, fingertips, mucous membranes of the lips and the genitals which respond poorly or not at all. In case the hair in the leucoderma lesions have become white, the chances of their repigmentation are very less. It is, however, not necessary that the non-hairy areas or the hairy areas with white hair would not repigment at all.

Sometimes, repigmentation starts from the periphery of the leucoderma patch, as the melanocytes progressively move inwards from the adjoining normal skin into the leucoderma patch. Occasionally, especially when the patches are recent and small, the entire patch may fade away completely.

For accurate assessment of the response to the treatment it is very essential to keep photographic records of all the lesions for an objective assessment, whether the lesions are increasing in size, have become static or have started getting repigmented. Without photographic records it may be very difficult to observe minor changes in the size of the lesions.

The photographs should be taken before starting the treatment and repeated at 2-4 months interval, especially for lesions that have shown improvement during this period. In case the lesions are large or multiple, the different regions should be photographed separately, so that different parts of the lesions can be compared area-wise for repigmentation or extension of the lesions.

CHAPTER

9 Surgical Treatment

Surgical treatment is needed as some patients are likely to be left with few lesions or part of lesion that do not develop repigmentation, irrespective of whatever treatment is given. Lesions located on the finger-tips, palms and soles, malleoli and the lips, and occasionally at other locations are likely to remain unpigmented in spite of treatment. If the lesions are located at cosmetically unimportant areas, they may be left alone. In case an unpigmented leucoderma lesion is situated on an exposed area or if the patient is keen to remove all lesions of leucoderma, such lesions can be subjected to surgical treatment. It is extremely important to ensure that the disease has become completely inactive before surgery is done. Otherwise, the disease can become active again and the surgically treated areas can also become depigmented leading to a great deal of frustration in the patient. There are no absolute criteria to ensure that the disease has indeed become inactive, except for the clinical judgement that the lesions are neither increasing nor decreasing in size or number for the last 6 months atleast. The longer the duration of inactivity in the lesions, the greater the certainty that the disease has indeed become inactive. The various surgical methods used for treating leucoderma include.

SPLIT-THICKNESS SKIN GRAFTING

This technique was first used for treating residual leucoderma lesion(s) by an Indian skin specialist in 1973. The technique consists of removing a piece of skin consist of epidermis and the superficial

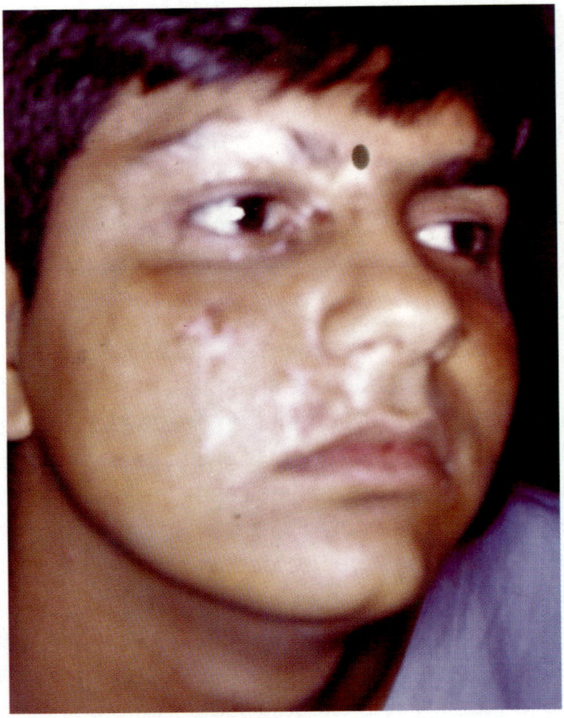

Fig. 9.1: Leucoderma face–before graft

portion of the dermis and transferring this sheet to the recipient vitiligo area which has been prepared by dermabrasion. The preparation of the recipient vitiligo area and the donor area is done by sterilization with savlon, spirit or povidone iodine scrubbing. If the area is hairy, it should be shaved. The dermabrasion is done with a motorized (electrical) or a manual dermabrader. The dermabraded area should include a narrow (2-3 mm) rim of the normal-looking surrounding skin also. The dermabrasion is carried out to the level of upper portion of the dermis (inner part of skin) till superficial pinpoint bleeding starts appearing. The area should be kept covered with moist gauze.

The donor skin is taken from the antero-lateral part of the thigh(s), the medial part of arm or the buttocks of the patient. A thin graft of superficial skin is taken by a sterile razor (shaving) blade or by a Humby's knife. The graft is then placed over the recipient area and fixed in place with collodion or by a proper pressure dressing. It is usual to leave an extra rim of donor skin, which is trimmed after 7 days when the dressing is opened to achieve complete coverage of the recipient area.

An alternative method of applying the graft consists of spreading the graft over vaseline gauze or Sofra-tulle (a type of dressing materials) cut to the shape and the size of the recipient area and placing the graft with the gauze on it. Stitching is generally not required. This method allows easy spreadability of the graft. Dressing is removed after 7-10 days. Antibiotics are preferably used for 7-10 days after the operation to prevent infection. This procedure requires

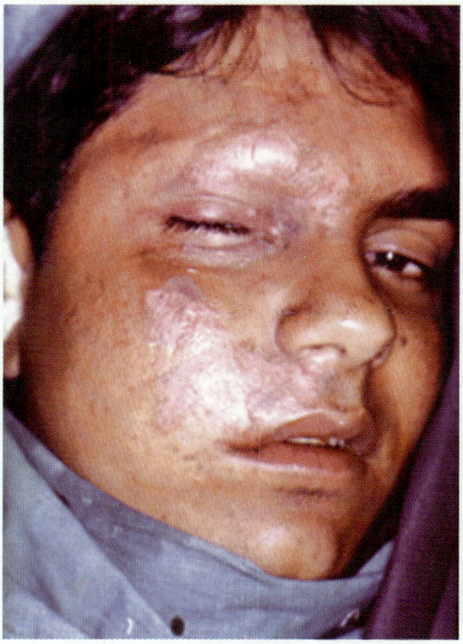

Fig. 9.2: Leucoderma face–immediately after split thickness graft

a complete surgical set-up. The complications of split thickness grafting include hyperpigmentation, hypertrophic scarring or keloid formation, graft rejection or peripheral depigmentation. These complications, however, are very infrequent and can be managed with appropriate treatment.

Complete color matching at the site of applying the graft and also the donor site may however, take a few months. The periphery of the old lesion may also remain visible for several months after the grafting.

The chief advantage of split thickness grafting is that even a large area can be covered in a single or at the most in a few sittings and there is no need to wait for the perigraft spread of the pigmentation.

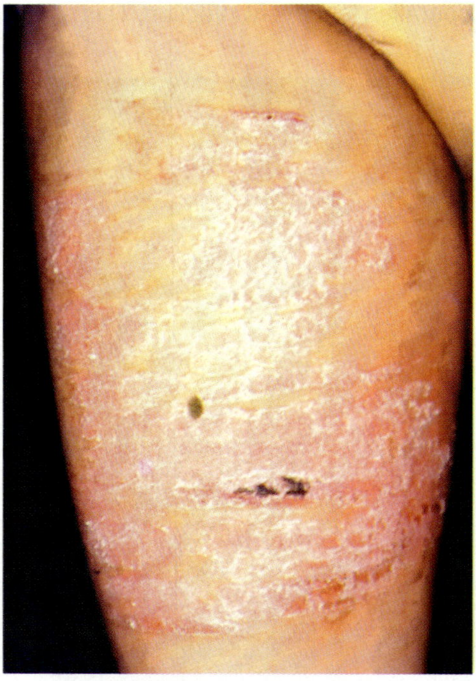

Fig. 9.3: Donor site in split graft after 2 weeks

SUCTION BLISTER GRAFTING

The procedure of skin grafting in leucoderma primarily involves transferring melanocytes from the pigmented skin areas to the leucoderma lesions. The melanocytes are present only in the epidermis. It should be enough to use sheets of epidermis for grafting over the leucoderma lesions. Sheets of normal epidermis can be obtained by using glass cups or funnels attached to a vacuum pump. A negative pressure of about 150 mm Hg leads to dermo-epidermal separation and the formation of a blister within 3-4 hours. The roof of the blister is snipped with a scissor and then applied on the recipient area prepared by dermabrasion and pressed over the area with a pad and tight bandage. Stitches are not required. The bandage is kept for seven days and the area prevented from getting wet. Systemic antibiotics can also be used during this period to prevent infection. At the end of seven days, the dressing can be removed. In this

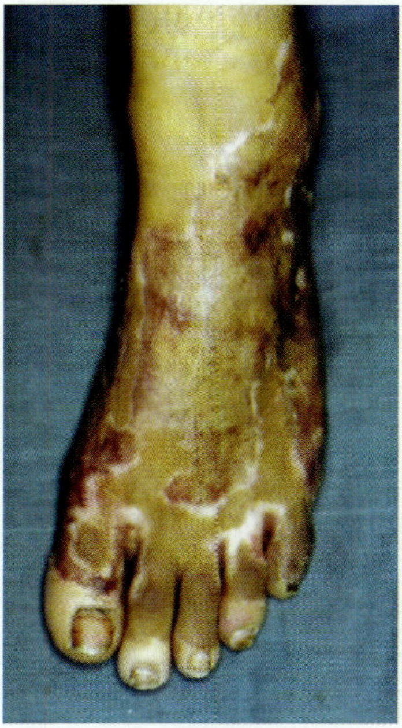

Fig. 9.4: Leucoderma feet–6 months after graft and shrinkage of graft as white area

procedure the entire area gets repigmented completely although the color match may not be perfect immediately. With time however, the color matching tends to improve. The chief disadvantages of this technique are: (1) it is a time consuming procedure, (2) the blister is painful; and (3) occasionally the patient may develop haematoma at the recipient site. This technique is however useful for smaller lesions.

PUNCH GRAFTING

This is a very simple technique that consists of transplanting pieces of normal skin obtained from a donor site with the help of a skin biopsy punch to the recipient leucoderma areas after removing the affected skin with a slightly smaller size biopsy punch. The sizes of punches usually used by various workers vary from 1.5 to 3 mm for recipient site and usually 0.5 mm larger for the donor sites.

The usual donor areas are the buttocks, the thighs or the medial side of the arms. The sites have to be prepared with savlon, spirit or

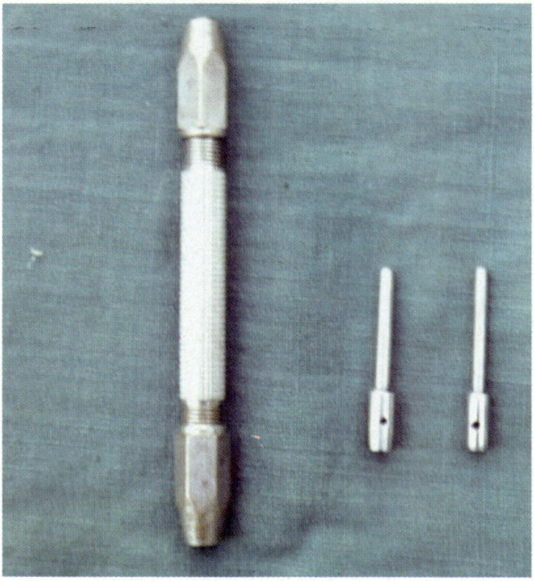

Fig. 9.5: Punches and handle

povidone iodine or with any other standard method of scrubbing and sterilization. Local anaesthesia with 2% xylocaine with or without adrenaline depending upon the site is given. After the surgery, the donor area is dressed with a pressure bandage after applying a vaseline gauze or Sofra-tulle. The grafts in the recipient area are also held in position by a similar pressure dressing for a week or so.

The major limitation of this technique is the time taken for complete repigmentation of the entire lesion. In addition, the grafted skin is usually visible in the patch for prolong period, although with time the grafts tend to merge with surrounding skin. In case, the grafted skin projects out of the general surface of the skin, the projected portion of the graft can be shaved off.

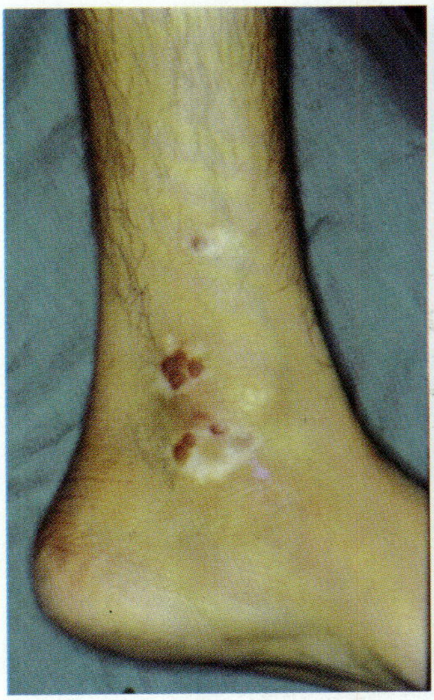

Fig. 9.6: Punch graft–pigmentation after 6 months

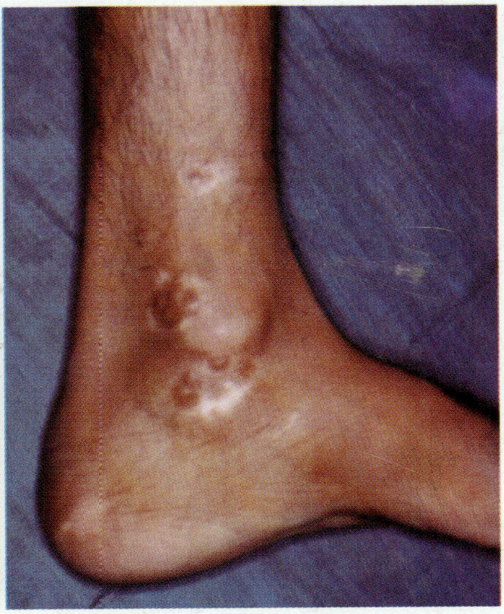

Fig. 9.7: Punch graft–pigmentation after 1 year

Sometimes, the pigmented areas around the grafts do not merge with each other, producing a cobblestone appearance. This however, is a temporary phase. The skin color tends to become homogenous with time.

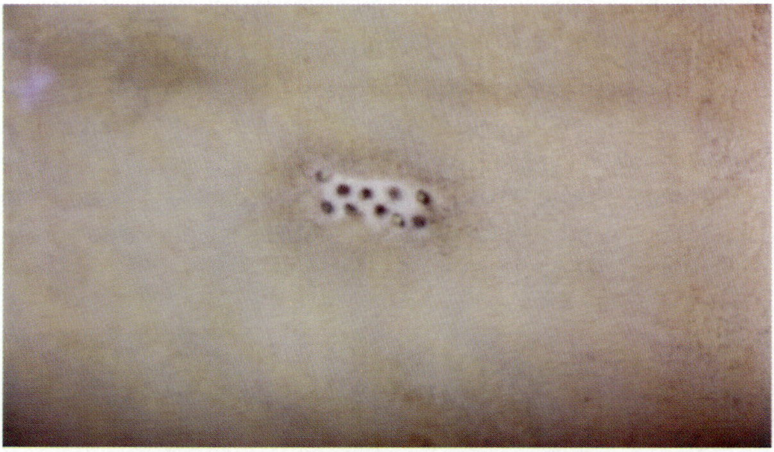

Fig. 9.8: Punch graft–donor site after 1 week

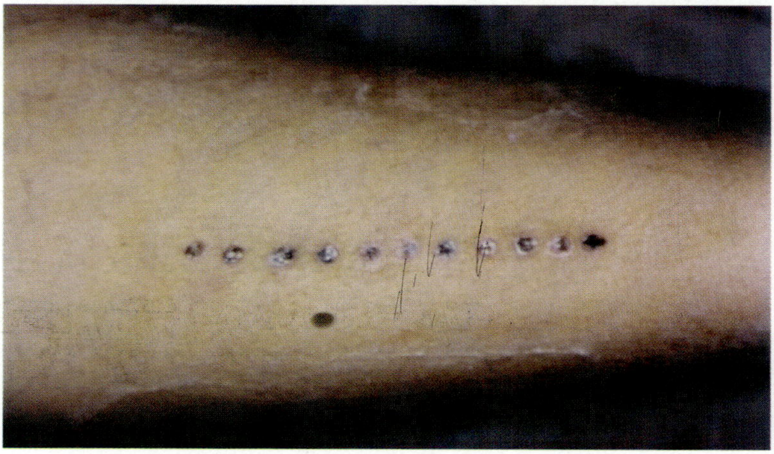

Fig. 9.9: Punch graft–donor site after 2 weeks

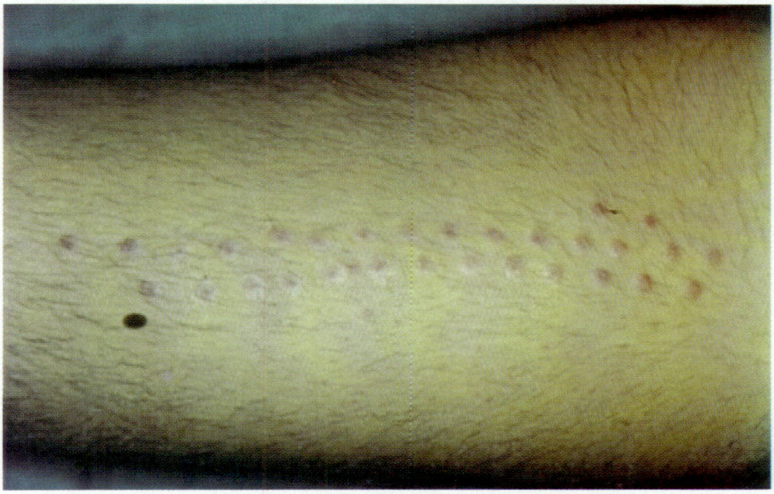

Fig. 9.10: Punch graft–donor site after 6 months

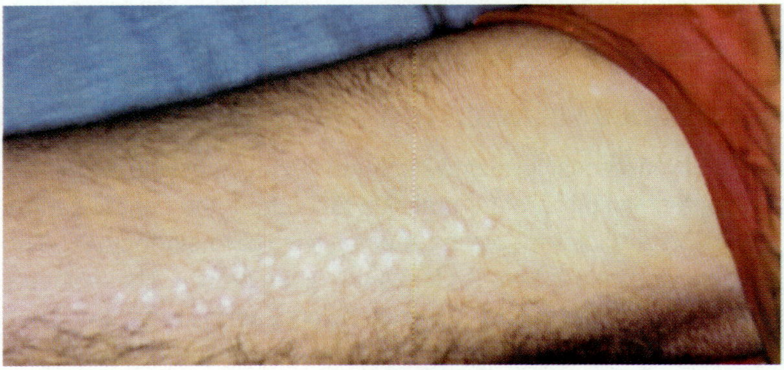

Fig. 9.11: Punch graft–donor site after 1 year

In addition, some of the punch grafts may not take because of infection and/or exudation under the skin graft or damage to the grafted skin by mishandling during the operation.

This risk can be minimized by taking appropriate care during the procedure.

HAIR FOLLICLE GRAFTING

Single hair follicle grafting is another method for repigmentation of leucoderma area especially if it has white hair (leucotrichia). Hair are taken from back of the head (occipital) and grafted on the leucoderma patch. It is a very simple and easy procedure. The color usually appears on the white patch by 4th or 5th week after single hair grafting as compare to 3rd week with other procedures. The color match is more acceptable than the color produced after other methods.

MESH GRAFTING

This method of grafting is used when large area of leucoderma need to be grafted and the pigmented skin area (donor site) is limited. In this, donor skin is enlarged to cover a large body surface. By meshing skin is enlarged by passing through a machine which makes small slits which on expansion make the skin like fish net. The size of mesh varies in ratio from 1:1 to 1:6. Following mesh grafting color (pigment) occurs in the space between the mesh which fills in with new skin growth.

AUTOLOGOUS MELANOCYTE GRAFTING

Since it is now possible to grow (culture) the melanocytes on artificial media, a small piece of normal skin taken from the patient can be grown on artificial media by multiplying the melanocytes. The melanocytes take 2-5 weeks for an adequate growth. These sheets can then be transferred to the recipient leucoderma areas that have been prepared by dermabrasion. This procedure needs a well equipped laboratory. At present it is still costly.

SURGICAL EXCISION OF THE LESION

In case the residual leucoderma lesion is very small, a simple surgical excision of the entire lesion may be all that is needed. In such cases, it is necessary to ensure that the scar after excision is as small and inconspicuous as possible.

CHAPTER

10 Camouflaging the White Patches

Since leucoderma is chiefly a cosmetic problem and the recovery with treatment is slow, many patients want to camouflage their lesions even as the treatment is continuing. This is especially required when the patient has to attend some social functions/occasions. A camouflage means hiding the lesion. Camouflage can be done by covering the area with a suitable cream, which has a color matching with the color of the skin of the patient. Such creams are made by mixing opaque agents with toning agents of red, yellow, brown and black color in different proportions to produce creams of various shades. Since the color of individuals belonging to different races vary widely, it is necessary to produce a large variety of shades to match the complexion of various individuals. However, such creams should be inert and non-sensitizing; and as far as possible should not get removed during sweating or getting drenched in the rain or while swimming. Such creams are usually easily washable with soap. Therefore, application of the cream is needed every time the area is washed. The cream is also likely to stain the clothes.

The lesion can also be camouflaged by applying henna paste. It is prepared by drying the leaves of henna (Lawsonia alba) plant and crushing them to obtain a powder. This powder is mixed with water to form a paste, which is applied on the lesion(s). Staining is obtained in 2-4 hours, though shorter duration of application will produce lighter color. The stain obtained is of a yellowish red color, which does not exactly match the skin color of most people. Washing the skin with an alkaline soap leads to darkening of the color. The stain lasts for a week or so.

Staining of the skin lesion can also be obtained by applying a concentrated aqueous solution of potassium permanganate over the leucoderma patch. The staining is instantaneous. The depth of the color can be adjusted by using an appropriate concentration of potassium permanganate. The color match with the surrounding skin is better. The stain is resistant to water and sweat but it does not last more than 24 hours.

Application of silver nitrate solution on the skin also produces a brownish black stain, which can last for several days, depending upon the concentration of silver nitrate in the solution. This concentration can vary between 1-5% to obtain the desired color, but silver nitrate generally produces very dark shades with a poor color match.

TATTOOING

This is another method of camouflage in which an opaque dye either of a black color or a mixture of red, yellow, black and brown are deposited in the superficial dermis to compensate for the absence of melanin. The dyes have got to be inert so that the tissues do not react to the dyes.

Tattooing should be used only as a last resort, and only for the residual leucoderma lesions as an alternative to the surgery. It must be ensured that the disease has really become inactive.

The main drawback of tattooing is that one can still make out that the skin in this region is not normal.

DEPIGMENTING THE PIGMENTED AREA

Patients who develop extensive leucoderma and decide not to take any treatment, often prefer to have a uniformly depigmented skin. They are unhappy if there are small residual areas of normally pigmented skin, especially on the exposed parts like face, hands

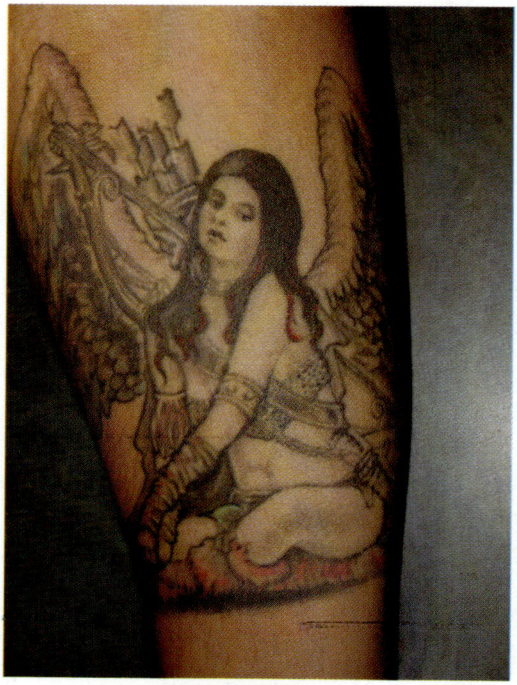

Fig. 10.1: Tattoo

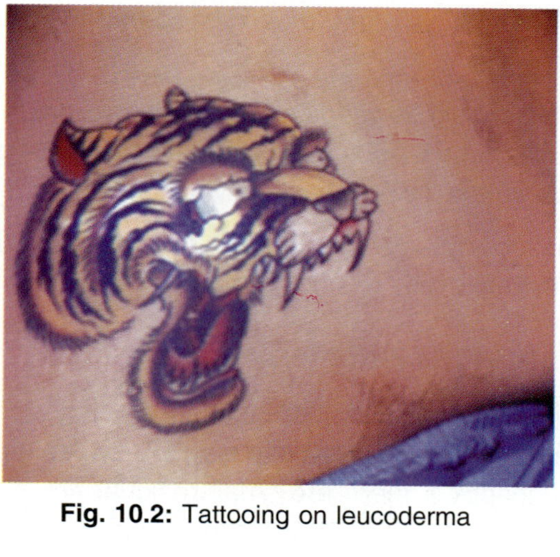

Fig. 10.2: Tattooing on leucoderma

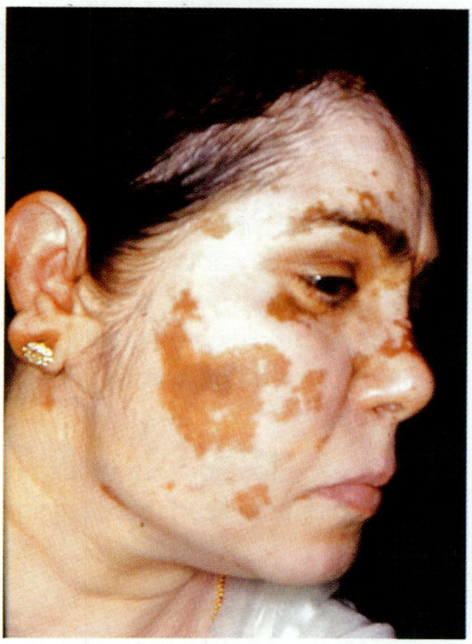

Fig. 10.3: Pigmentation on face in total leucoderma

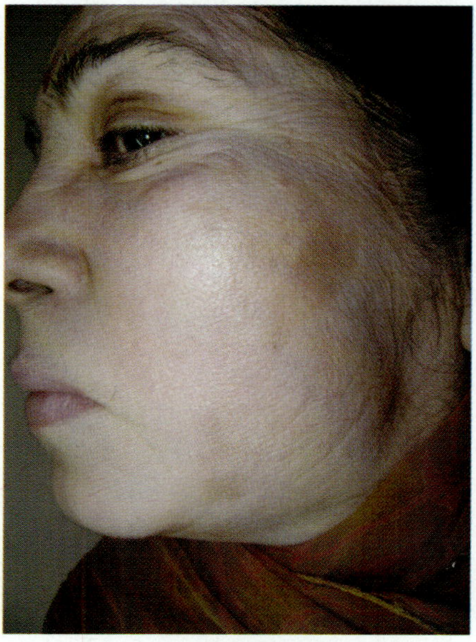

Fig. 10.4: Total leucoderma–face

and forearms. These areas due to routine day-to-day exposure to sunlight tend to stimulate repigmentation at these sites. To remove these patches of normally pigmented skin, the patient can be advised to use an ointment containing 20% monobenzyl ether of hydroquinone, a chemical used in the manufacturing of rubber, which has the potential of permanently destroying the melanocytes. One or two applications of this ointment per day can be continued till the areas of normally pigmented skin also become depigmented and the patient achieves a uniformly depigmented complexion. The action of the chemical is slow, takes 1-4 months to start and complete depigmentation may be achieved in 10-12 months.

The skin should be protected from sunlight with clothes or sunscreen because pigmentation can recur anytime.

CHAPTER

11 No Treatment of Leucoderma

Lastly, it is equally important to be aware that leucoderma is essentially an innocuous disease. Apart from the fact that the patient has an uneven distribution of skin color, he/she can be as efficient physically, mentally, sexually and intellectually as any other individual. A patient having leucoderma feels handicapped only because his colleagues, friends and relatives do not approve of the depigmented patches. If we realize that we do not mind dogs, cats, cows, buffaloes, tigers and all the other animals who have patches of different colors on their skin, we have no valid reason to reject a human being who does not have a uniform distribution of his/her skin color. The patient should therefore, be made to realize that they can decide not to take any treatment at all and live efficiently and happily in spite of leucoderma. The pigmented skin is only slightly more susceptible to sunlight and may require a bit more of protection, whenever one is overexposed to the sun.

It needs to be reiterated that patients having leucoderma have no abnormality other than the loss of the pigment. In all other functions, they are absolutely normal. It is therefore acceptable for a person to choose to take no treatment for leucoderma. This decision may be taken by an individual who primarily feels that there is no need for treatment. More commonly however, a person may decide to take no treatment or give up treatment because he/she thinks that it involves too much of an effort, or because he/she is disappointed with the results. He/she may also give up the treatment when the disease becomes inactive. Some patients may not take the treatment because they are not aware that an effective treatment is available, while some others may not know the treatment or give it up because they are misled into believing that the treatment is toxic or ineffective. When a patient decides not to take the treatment, this should be an informed decision. However, if such a decision is based on misconceptions and misbelieves, it is the duty of the concerned skin specialist to provide the correct information.

CHAPTER

12

Conclusion

With this information it should be obvious that leucoderma can now be treated in almost all the cases. The patients who do not recover are often to be blamed themselves. There are a large variety of therapeutic measures available for treating this disease, one can therefore select the procedure most suitable for the patient, but if a patient does not respond to one therapeutic procedure, he/she should be treated with an alternate procedure. It is also necessary to evaluate the response to treatment from time to time so that the procedure can be modified whenever it becomes necessary to do so. The treatment has to be continued till one can be reasonably certain that the disease has disappeared completely and there is no chance for the disease to become active again.

An attempt must be made to ensure that all the lesions get repigmented or are removed with or without surgical intervention. In any case, it should be the patient who should have the final say for deciding whether she/he wants to have any treatment at all. Needless to say, that the earlier the treatment is started the better is the end result.

The patients who allow themselves to be misguided by unscrupulous and non-scientific advices are likely to end up in disaster and should consider themselves to be responsible for the consequences of their decision.

INDEX